HOWARD, STANLEY, AND ME

Howard, Stanley, and Me

A Long Journey with Cancer

By

WILLIAM D. AND GAIL M. MAYO

XULON PRESS

Xulon Press
2301 Lucien Way #415
Maitland, FL 32751
407.339.4217
www.xulonpress.com

Unless otherwise indicated, Scripture quotations taken from the King James Version (KJV)—*public domain.*

Printed in the United States of America.

ISBN-13: 978-1-6305-0449-6

In remembrance:

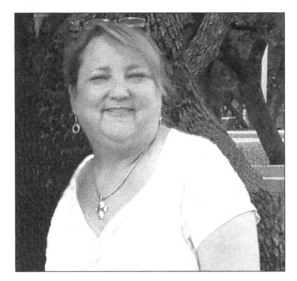

Cynthia Lorraine Roth

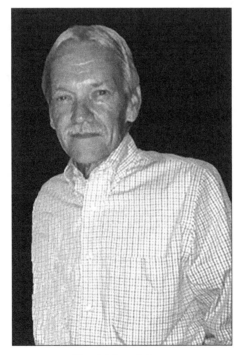

David Lee Mayo

Contributing Author:

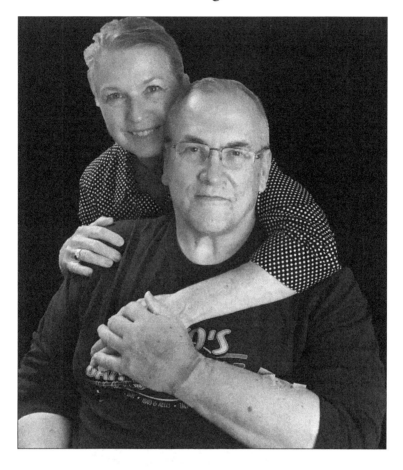

Gail is respected and admired as a consummate home-maker, wife, mother, and grandmother. Howard, Stanley, and Me is her first writing project as a contributing author. She has long been encouraged by her husband and kids to write; as she definitely has something to say and is worth listening to. She is artistic in many areas – from decorating, to gardening, to gourmet cuisine, music, and watercolor painting. She is mom to five kids and grandma to seventeen grandkids. And most notably, a trusted advisor and counselor to one hard headed husband.

About the Illustrator:

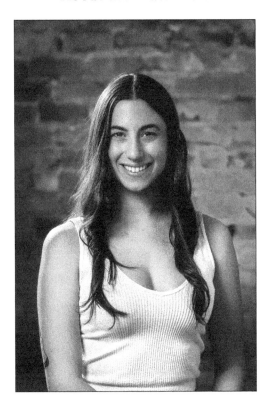

Jessica was born in Georgetown, DC, and received her BFA from James Madison University with a concentration in drawing and painting. She is currently working on painting and illustration in Richmond, Virginia.

"I love rendering the human form, exploring surreal illustration, and creating meticulous drawings. When reading the author's intimate account of his journey with cancer, what stood out to me most was his brazen positivity and the incredible impact hope and his faith has had in helping him persevere. The bottom banner of the cover is my artistic rendering of spindle cell sarcoma cancer and the swallow rising out of the dark symbolizes the author's triumph - carried up through the wings of hope."

FOREWORD

BY

DR. ROB PRESCOTT

I met my friend Bill Mayo over seventeen years ago in the summer of 2002, when he was in charge of the Track-Type Tractor Division of Caterpillar, Inc., a Fortune-50 company known almost everywhere in the world for their earth-moving, mining, and power equipment and in England for their boots.

Bill had decided to pursue a master's degree in English at that time because he knew the importance of writing, not only because of his leadership role at Caterpillar but because he had so much to say about the things that mattered most to him as a human being—as a son, a brother, a husband, a father, and a grandfather.

On the one hand, he knew that interpersonal communication skills were vital to his success in business, but on the other, and more importantly, he wanted to find a way to express important things—spiritual and ethical issues—in ways that would reach the people who could genuinely benefit from them.

Bill then left Bradley for a few years to supervise CAT Europe East and West, but he kept working on his master's degree the whole time. When he returned to the U.S. as vice-president of Cat's North American Commercial Division, he completed a screenplay centered around one of the pivotal questions he found the most compelling: "What is the opposite of faith? Is it doubt, or is it certainty?" Spoiler alert—it's certainty.

That film, *Out of the Heart*, is now available to anyone on Amazon Prime, directed by his son Michael with original music by his son Bob. That film, like this book, is a hallmark of Bill's character—when he has something to say, he finds a way to say it. When he takes on a challenge, he finishes it.

This book is an after-action report about the greatest challenge Bill ever faced, and he wants to share with you everything he learned along the way. He is not cautioning anyone here about how *not* to cope with life-threatening cancer. Far from it. Instead, he hopes to share with everyone involved—the patient, the spouses, the children, the friends, the doctors, the nurses and nurse's aides—that for him, the affirmative strength to endure was found in his complete surrender to God.

As you will see, Bill fought with "Stanley," his highly unusual and highly aggressive cancer, as intensely as Ahab fought with the white whale. While he filmed *Out of the Heart*, in fact, he was still in a pitched battle with just one of the cancer's recurrences. Yet Stanley kept coming back, in spite of all the hardship Bill and his family endured to fight and fight and fight, day after day for over eight years.

This book is a narrative roller-coaster in which Bill shares the ups and downs, from the heights of horror and despair as the cancer recurred again and again to the various ways that God (known to us now as "Howard") somehow hopped into the seat next to Bill and rode with him down to a condition of enlightened peace.

With each version of Stanley, then, the peace at the end of the ride was more complete, more clear, and more confident—and best of all, contagious.

For all those who have suffered severe medical challenges, you will see that Bill's moments of greatest insight mirror your own, in that they were mediated by family and friends who love him. Bill's healing, in all its dimensions, did not come in a vacuum.

God touched him through his wife Gail, through his children and grandchildren, through his doctors and caregivers, and through his friends.

He made his decision to choose a radical solution to his cancer, as so many do, not for himself but for Gail and for all who love him. That love led him to willingly part with his entire right leg rather than see his loved ones continue to fear that Stanley would return one more time.

In the early chapters of the book, we see Bill struggling with the onset of his fight with Stanley, always with the power of his good humor yet without the power to win the battle. But there are turning points. The first came when he realized he could not put Gail through another round of cancer. The second was when his daughter Erin helped him understand that in losing his leg, he had not been diminished. Their love freed him to be at peace at exactly the right moment, and this is how it is for all who endure life-threatening disease—God comes to us, not "trailing clouds of glory" but in the simple acts and words of love.

Bill Mayo wrote this book not only for those battling cancer but for those who fight alongside them, to help everyone see the many ways in which prayer lifts the patient up and makes the medicinal power of grace more potent.

For anyone who has not been a part of such a fight with cancer, this book opens a window into that experience and is thus a priceless chance to grow in understanding and compassion. That sounds complicated, but it's really important. We all need to grow in our capacity for prayer, especially when those we love face cancer and we don't know what to say or do.

It takes us beyond that struggle, however, to Bill's enduring sense of peace and confidence, his sense of gratitude, and his appreciation for all the good things in his life. These in turn allow him to cope with the "phantom pain" that very few of us will ever experience and thus fully understand. We see, too, that once his final surgery was complete, he was supported by others who experienced the same thing, with the same optimism and gratitude we see in Bill.

Howard, Stanley, and Me is a book worth sharing with anyone touched by cancer—not simply because it is a tale of victory but because it is a funny, emotionally moving, and painfully real example of how an ordinary person can find healing by surrendering humbly to God and trusting in the love of family and friends.

TABLE OF CONTENTS

Prologue xv

1. Cast of Characters 1
2. Introducing Stanley 5
3. Introducing Me 11
4. Introducing Howard 17
5. Stanley – Up Close and Personal 21
6. Houston, We Have a Problem. 25
7. Me, Up Close and Personal. 33
8. Howard, Up Close and Personal. 47
9. M.D. Anderson vs. Stanley – Take One 71
10. M.D. Anderson vs. Stanley – Take Two 77
11. M.D. Anderson vs. Stanley – Third Time's the Charm. 81
12. Home Again, Home Again – Jiggity-Jig. 97
13. Introducing Gail 101

Epilogue 111

PROLOGUE

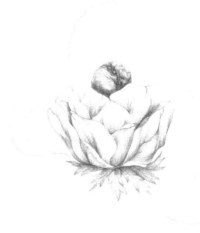

W elcome to my story—the story of my personal journey with cancer. To be precise, my journey with Stage III, undifferentiated, pleomorphic spindle-cell sarcoma of the right thigh.

Most stories, I suppose, begin at the beginning. That's logical enough, but I actually struggled with identifying the precise onset of my story. Frankly, I'm not sure when the beginning began!

Historically, cancer is nothing new in my family. My father died of cancer at fifty-nine. My mother died of cancer at seventy-three. My brother died of cancer at sixty-eight. My grandparents on both sides and several aunts and uncles also succumbed to the *Big C*. There is a lot of cancer history in the family, but I've learned that history matters little when it comes to traveling your own road with this disease. It is uniquely personal.

In my history, I was diagnosed with cancer over eight years ago. I am not at the beginning of my journey. Cancer has been with me for a while now. I also know with certainty that the journey is not yet over. There is always a risk of recurrence. Or it can pop up somewhere else. One never knows.

I do suspect I'm well beyond half-time of this journey—although, of course, I can't quantitatively prove it. But considering I'm currently sixty-seven years old, cancer or no cancer, I'm in the fourth quarter of life with the clock ticking down toward the buzzer. I'm not yet deceased, so clearly (and thankfully) I've not yet reached the end of my life's story. So, let's just say that I'm somewhere on my own timeline—unsure when it precisely began or when it will end. I only know where I'm at in the moment—in the present. Thus, the present is where I'll begin.

And at this very moment, the *present* is defined as a bed in a hotel room across the street from the M.D. Anderson Cancer Center in Houston, Texas. The year is 2019. It's a little after 2:00 am. I was discharged from the cancer center a week ago (June 27th) to spend some time recovering away from the germ incubator known as a hospital.

While arguably better than being cooped up in a hospital, I'm still cooped up. I find myself lying here for a good majority of each day and night—staring at the ceiling—trying to get my mind around what happened just one week ago on Thursday, June 20th, 2019. I know what happened, of course. But knowing and embracing that truth are two distinctly different things.

So, what happened? It was a nifty yet complex five-and-a-half-hour surgical procedure known in the orthopedic community as a total hip disarticulation amputation. In other words, I have no right leg from the hip joint down. My right side ends rather abruptly at a butt cheek.

The team of physicians at M.D. Anderson Cancer Center removed my entire leg—all because of a measly ten inches of tumor encasing my sciatic nerve and femoral artery. Earlier treatments over the course of the prior eight years included twenty-eight days of intense chemotherapy, twenty-five days of radiation, and two prior tumor resections. None of those efforts killed the little bugger. (Although *little* is a relative term, as the first tumor actually weighed in at a reasonably hefty two-and-a-half pounds!) The second tumor was only about the size of an adult fist. And, as I said, the third recurrence was about ten inches in length—a spidery little bugger with fingers extending into various cavities of my thigh. This cancer was proving itself a persistent and stubborn tumor that appeared to really enjoy its accommodation in my right leg.

I've gotten used to this tumor being with me over the past eight years—life goes on. I've been continually aware of the constant threat of recurrence. After surgery number one, total eradication wasn't achieved because of its proximity to the sciatic nerve and the femoral artery. I learned about *margins* after surgery number one.

Margins are the distance between cancerous tissue removed and the good tissue that remains. Negative margins are a good thing. Positive margins are not. When no cancer cells are detected at the outer edge of the removed tissue, that's a negative margin—a good result. When cancer cells extend into the edge of the removed tissue sample, that's a positive margin—and not what you want to hear. After the first two tumor resections, I heard the same result—positive margins. How ironic that a *positive result* has such negative impact!

As they say, however, the third time's the charm. For margins, that is. The tumor recurred once again in the same location—right posterior thigh—but this time with a decidedly nasty attitude. He was now growing quite a bit faster and was actually encasing key vascular and nerve structures within my leg, affecting both mobility and sensation. The tumor also retained one of its most stubborn qualities...it would not respond to chemo or radiation.

There's a good deal to think about while staring at ceilings in the early morning or late night hours. Chief among them was the lingering thought that I had walked into the hospital fully ambulatory, while knowing that to manage this disease, I would eventually leave the hospital unable to walk. Yes, the margins were now negative. But so was my leg. It was gone.

It's counterintuitive to think that a cure meant losing a perfectly good leg. My doctors—two wonderful women named Dr. Valerae Lewis and Dr. Alysia Kemp—described my decision to amputate as a "difficult but courageous and brave decision." I heard them say more than once, "It was the wise choice." Presumably because it would, indeed, remove cancer from my body. *Life over limb,* they affirmed. Amputation would finally achieve the negative margins desired. But there's the rub, right? Without cancer, I would not be able to walk. With cancer, I was just days ago still fully ambulatory.

Yeah, I'll admit it. It was more than mildly surreal to get my head around the concept of being an amputee before the surgery. It's certainly surreal post-surgery as well. Still today, my mind does loops around the irony. ***I could walk with cancer. I am crippled without it.*** But there is a greater message here. And although darkened ceilings don't highlight those lessons well, I anticipate that as I unpack this experience in the chapters that follow, throughout the chronicle of my personal journey, the lessons will become more clear. I invite you to join me in the discovery.

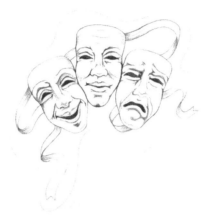

CAST OF CHARACTERS

For now, as I've said, I'm still wrapping my head around the fact that my leg is no longer present. I fret about future mobility. I fret even more about loss of independence. There are everyday reminders of this new reality, of course. Things like how long it takes to get up from bed or just to turn *in* bed. How long it takes to hobble with a walker to the restroom in the middle of the night. Reminders of the necessity to sometimes contort my body to avoid sitting on a large plastic drain in my right side. Reminders that I haven't had a full-on shower in two weeks, and sponge baths just don't cut it. Reminders of how difficult it can be to sit on a toilet seat. And reminders known as phantom limb pain (PLP), which is excruciating pain in a limb that is no longer a part of my body.

Beyond those all-too-real reminders, embracing the truth of what happened and why it happened to me is the story of this book. Most people question why God allows bad things to happen to so-called *good* people. In my personal passage, I believe I do know the **why**. And beyond the **why**, I can also see the **how**. And I feel I should share that beyond myself.

To do so, to explain this to a casual observer, requires exploring my timeline along with three primary characters. I should point out it's actually a cast of hundreds if not thousands of people who walked this journey with me. But for purposes of explaining what and how it all happened, it's primarily a cast of three. And I'd like you to meet them.

The first character you'll meet is Stanley. Stanley is the name my grandchildren first conferred upon my cancerous tumor. Both the first tumor which officially arrived following discovery of a suspicious lump in July 2011 and Stanley's so-called cousins, First Cousin Stanley in July of 2017 and Second Cousin Stanley in April of 2019. Why Stanley? We'll get to that. But it was simply a name that stuck.

The second character you'll meet is me. Now I've always said that we are each three people—who we think we are, who we want others to think we are, and who we really are. I've also suggested that the journey of one's life is to integrate those three perceptions into one whole being. I think I would define maturity as the point at which who we are is ideally the homogeneous blend of each perception. In this story, you'll meet all three Me's.

The final character in this journey is the most important. And that's Howard. Howard is my physician. He's also my friend. He's so instrumental to this journey, I anticipate even as I am writing this now that I will do a poor job explaining His multi-faceted role. But I'll give it a shot. Anyway, Howard is key, and I'm eager to share His impact with each reader.

Obviously, there are hundreds more people involved with my journey, past, present, and future. Wonderful nurses, exceptional physicians, nursing assistants, physical therapists, occupational therapists, prosthetists, family, and dear friends. It isn't fair to reduce my story to just three characters, I know. With profound thanks, I am humbly grateful to each and every one whose thumb-prints are on this story—and upon me. Many have touched me in ways they will never fully realize, and I thank each person from the bottom of my heart.

In the telling of this tale, with apologies to those many others, I will relate my story about a rather stubborn and relentless tumor named Stanley, an incomplete and evolving me, and a wonderful physician named Howard. It's been a fabulous journey thus far, and I'm fully aware that it's not over. Still, it's sufficiently far along for me to tell what needs to be told. And with that as introduction, I begin.

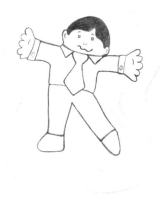

INTRODUCING STANLEY

I'm not sure when Stanley first took up residence in my right thigh. No idea, actually. My first introduction to Stanley occurred in June of 2011 in the Big Apple. He wasn't named Stanley at this point, however. He was just a lump. His name came much later. I was introduced to, shall I say *it*, at that time—it being defined as a rather large, hard mass in my right posterior thigh.

I had been in New York for a board meeting earlier in the week, and my wife, Gail, flew out from Illinois on June 8th to join me for a long weekend in the city. We were celebrating our thirty-seventh wedding anniversary in style—staying in a Times Square hotel in downtown Manhattan, seeing some great shows, going to a comedy club, and eating great food, not to mention merely soaking up the energy of the city that never sleeps. We were having a great time, and even though the city never sleeps, we slept in on Saturday, June 11th. This was going to be our last day before flying back home to Illinois, and we were content just vegging from packing in so much on Thursday and Friday. It was to be a lazy morning. We were sitting up in bed, both reading the newspaper. I had the paper propped against my knees. Gail was in essentially the same position adjacent to me, and we were enjoying a relaxing pre-breakfast respite.

At some point, I shifted the paper to turn the page and noticed for the first time a rather prominent lump on the back of my leg. I looked at it for a moment. I thought it was nothing— perhaps just the way I was propping up my leg. I stretched my leg out straight, and sure enough, it was still there. Actually, it looked even larger in that position. Finally, convinced that this *nothing* was actually *something*, I said out loud, "What in the heck is *that*?"

Gail lowered her section of the paper and looked over to see what I had made such a big deal about. She said something both humorous and profound. "Bill, that doesn't look right. You need to get that checked." She positioned herself a little better to examine this lump and was convincing with her description—it was a pronounced, large, and unyielding mass.

Truth be told, I had never noticed it before. I never had any symptoms, and despite its unusual existence, for me it was nothing to become alarmed about. Or at least I chose to discount any distress. Still, after pressing and probing on it for a while myself, I concluded (with Gail's strong encouragement) that it wasn't to be ignored.

Now, I'm not making excuses, but I guess it comes with the territory of being a *typical guy.* I made an appointment to see my family physician two months later. I know, way to get right on it, right? Don't think for a moment that Gail wasn't pressing me to take action. She was. But I always found something—anything and many things—to take precedence over making a doctor's appointment. I finally did so in August of 2011.

My family doc at the time wasn't too alarmed. He questioned any potential trauma, of course, and there had been none. He suggested that perhaps the best course of action would be to get an MRI. So, on September 6th, 2011, I got my first of many MRIs. I was to call my family doc a few days later, which I did. (Applause for punctuality inserted here!) My doc said the reading looked like a hematoma—fancy word for a bruise. He said it also looked to the radiologist as if there might be some kind of fluid build-up—which further suggested a hematoma—a collection of blood under the skin. He thought it would eventually go down and re-absorb into the body, so nothing to worry about. Great news!

Since Gail and I were soon to fly to England for a wedding, I asked the only relevant question I could think of at the moment—"Can I fly with this?" He responded in the affirmative, and not long thereafter, we had a great trip to England. In fact, life went on pretty much as normal. We traveled; we had adventures; we had lots of good family time. My boys and I were even launching a new creative adventure, trying to tackle movie production. Life was busy, and life was good. I participated normally, accompanied by a large (and seemingly to me), growing lump on the back of my leg. Gail remained freaked out.

In May of 2012, I decided (interpret that as Gail encouraged me) to get that lump checked out again, because contrary to my doc's prediction, the apparent fluid did not reabsorb into the body, and, in fact, that lump seemed even larger still. So, I saw the family doc on May 9th, 2012. He agreed it might be a little bigger and scheduled me for a second MRI.

About a month later, June 12th, I had that second MRI. Of course, the techs aren't allowed to tell you anything, but I will admit to sensing some sort of concerned look on her face. Still, I was able to put it out of my mind—even though the not knowing was driving Gail a bit nuts. That and what she perceived to be my cavalier attitude! A few days later, I got a call from my family doctor. I remember him saying really only one thing.

"Bill, there is *interval growth* from the September MRI to this latest one."

I asked, "Well, what's that mean?"

The doc explained it in a simple phrase: "It means I want you to go see a surgeon."

That seemed a big leap to me, but I asked him if he had someone in mind. He gave me the name of a fine local surgeon and informed me that he'd already set up the referral appointment. It's amazing how time can pile up on you while waiting for such things. My appointment with the surgeon was set for July 16th, 2012—another full month later. As a nervous Gail pointed out, a full month-plus from being notified that my current family doc didn't know what it was and had referred me to a general surgeon for evaluation. She was honked.

Nevertheless, I went to that appointment and immediately liked the surgeon. He was affable yet direct. He performed a cursory exam and said, "Well, Bill, it could be a cyst of some type, and I could remove it for you—but what's concerning is the interval growth." There was that phrase again—*interval growth*. It sounds so innocuous. Something got bigger from one point in time to the next. Still, Gail and I knew what they were implying without the *Big C* reference ever being spoken. The surgeon scheduled a biopsy for me. That occurred on July 25th, 2012.

I recall during the biopsy that the first needle used to penetrate Stanley actually broke. *Hard and fixed,* I remember thinking. Not a good sign in my mind. My friendly Internet had told me that "hard and fixed" was not a good thing. Finally, they got the biopsy sample, and I returned home to await the results. I suspected with some certainty what those results would be.

On August 2nd, 2012, my family doctor called to deliver the news. "Bill, I'm sorry, but you have cancer."

A full year following discovery of my New York lump, we finally called out the beast. I can't say I was surprised or devastated or otherwise shocked. I was pretty stoic, actually, as is my nature. The only thought I had was how I wanted to tell my kids, their spouses, and my grandkids—all thirteen of them. (By the way, today there are seventeen grandkids, and they are the joy of my life.) So, Gail and I discussed our approach, me opting for a text or email, she opting for a family dinner. We had a family dinner. (She always wins.)

Family gatherings are a relatively common occurrence for the Mayo household, so I'm quite sure no one was alarmed at another invitation. We had our gathering, and without much fanfare or drama, I simply told the kids the results of the biopsy and discussed next steps. My kids were great—three daughters (Erin, Macy, and Molly) and two sons (Mike and Bob)— all were very positive and encouraging, as were their spouses. The grandkids were also great and very curious. Because Gail and I were calm and not freaking out, neither were any of them. The grandkids wanted to know a bit more about what a tumor was, and in my explanation, I referred to it as *he*.

This naturally elicited their next question, "What's his name?"

I think it was my son-in-law Eric who first responded with, "Stanley."

Not sure where that came from, but one of the kids said, "Oh, like Flat Stanley?" And from that moment on, my tumor had its identity. We never talked tumor—we only talked Stanley.

Retrospectively, I think this was a brilliant accident! Namely, because it was a lot less frightening to talk about a stranger living in my leg named Stanley than it would have been to discuss the intimidating words *cancerous tumor*. Stanley also allowed us to have fun with him. Jokes about Stanley were routine. He became a guest of the family—albeit an unwelcome guest, perhaps—but a guest of the family that we simply hoped would eventually take his leave.

By the way, if you haven't heard of the Flat Stanley Project, it was a popular literacy project that millions of kids participated in around the world. The gist of the project was that *Flat Stanley*—a paper cut-out depiction of a little cartoon-like guy—was sent via mail to all sorts of people in innumerable places—relatives and friends, even celebrities around the world. The intended recipient would (hopefully) send Stanley back with a signature, maybe a picture, and the like. I think what appealed to my grandkids was the idea of sending Stanley packing. The only difference being, not one of us wanted to see him come back.

At least now with our unwelcome guest identified, it was time to figure out what to do to make him so uncomfortable that he would want to leave. The first step of that process took place on August 8th, 2012, at eleven o'clock in the morning. That was the day I first met an oncologist. My wife, oldest daughter Erin, and I went to Peoria's Illinois Cancer Care Center. We met the first of many cancer specialists. Her name was Dr. Jane Liu.

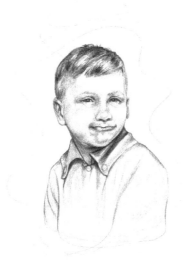

INTRODUCING ME

I am actually the least important character in this play, but I suppose you need to know a little about me since, after all, *me* is in the title of this tale!

I was born on January 8th, 1952. I'm thinking that's about all of my childhood you need to know in the retelling of this journey. For the mundanely curious, I was born in Pekin, Illinois. I graduated from Morton Illinois High School in 1970. I attended the U.S. Naval Academy and graduated in 1974. I served five years active duty and then sought to defy the author Thomas Wolfe—who wrote *You Can't Go Home Again*—and moved back to Morton. I also began working at Caterpillar Tractor Co. after taking a leave of three whole days upon discharge from the Navy. I stuck my wife with unpacking duties as we moved into our little Cape Cod home while I went about with commencement of my new career.

As I've already said, my father, mother, and brother all died of cancer at relatively young ages. My younger sister also passed, but she escaped *the Big C.* My father had always told us boys that no male relative in the Mayo clan ever lived passed sixty. He cited his grandfather, father, two brothers, and a number of distant relatives I never knew. So, I had a long history with cancer's impact on a family long before August 2nd, 2012.

With that as a brief personal history, I'll pick up the more intimate introduction to me at the point Dr. Liu informed us we would need to go to Houston to ensure a truly expert team would be focused on Stanley. Her humility in referring me was a bit surprising. She said Illinois Cancer Care saw about five cases a year of sarcoma-type cancers. She was new to Illinois Cancer Care but mentioned she had a good friend, a specialist in sarcoma, at M.D. Anderson—one of the country's leading cancer centers. She said M.D. Anderson treated nearly 100 cases of sarcoma-type cancers in a month. It was ironic that she was referring me to M.D. Anderson because when we'd received the diagnosis by phone from my family physician, we were hosting my dearest and best friend from high school and his wife at our home, Bob and Diane Cashen. Before the phone call with my doc, they had already been extolling the virtues of M.D. Anderson, a place I'd never heard of before. Bob and Diane heard the initial diagnosis within seconds of my phone call with the doc. Their prior suggestion of M.D. Anderson is just one of those interesting coincidences. A coincidence that, upon reflection, seemed to be directed by a higher power.

Although I appreciated Dr. Liu's willingness to play back-up to the experts, Houston was not a place I was particularly excited to return to. You see, Houston held awkward memories for me. After resigning my commission from the U.S. Navy in 1979, as I said, I joined the Midwest corporate giant Caterpillar Tractor Co. in its Marketing Training Program.

In that program, following six months of orientation and training, the first real assignment was to be a field representative's position. Now this was a coveted position for most young marketing types. But me? Well, I had already spent five years in the U.S. Navy, traveling around the world, being separated from my family. The last thing I wanted to do was take a position with a company that required relocation and travel. Ugh! What had I gotten myself into?

With an oceanography degree from the U.S. Naval Academy, Caterpillar was about my only employment option in town. I wasn't a college professor, so Bradley University was out. I wasn't a doctor, so the fine medical facilities in the Peoria area were out, too. In fact, the only company that would reasonably take a look at me was Caterpillar. I remember the company had a motto at the time: "To grow as fast in the future as we have in the past." I was still in the Navy when I first interviewed with them, and upon returning home to Great Lakes Naval Training Center following that initial interview in April of 1979, I remember telling Gail, "They're out of control, but they're having a good time."

I'm convinced that with my background, the **only** reason I got hired was because of this motto. I wouldn't cut it today in their environment, but at the time, they were willing to take a chance on a young, non-engineering-oriented guy because I had five years of military leadership experience. They intended to move people from their initial training and out into the field force as fast as possible. In fact, the first position they offered me after only four months was that coveted field service representative's position in (of all places) Houston, Texas.

I had a conflict. When I left the military and returned home to the Morton, Illinois, area, I truly just wanted to settle down. I didn't choose Caterpillar because I loved big machinery. I didn't choose marketing because I was an extroverted type. In fact, I really didn't realize I was hired *into* a marketing career path. How naïve was I? I chose Caterpillar because it was home.

All I knew in July of 1979 when I reported to work my first day was that I wanted to settle down. I wanted to stay put. And I wanted to get my life right in all ways—live a simple life with my wife and whatever family I was blessed with, have a small Cape Cod house with a white picket fence, and, basically, live my idealized vision of Ozzie & Harriett.

Part of getting that idealized vision right was getting my spiritual life right. In truth, shortly after I was hired onto Caterpillar, I began to repent of my past life and sins and was preparing to become a member of my local church and commit to Christ as a Christian believer. The last thing I wanted to do was move in the midst of this process.

When the offer was made, I said (not so confidently), "I'm not sure this is the right place for me to move." I didn't give my managers any reasons—at least not completely truthful reasons. I tried to slide out of this move without a lot of explanation. I was **so** naïve. I didn't know how corporations worked. Basically, it was the same as my previous employer, the United States Navy. They want you to go—and you go. Cheerfully. *You serve at the pleasure of the President,* we used to lament in the Navy. Well, my reluctance caused my employer, Caterpillar, to try a different approach. They thought that perhaps a little *get acquainted* visit to Houston would help to turn around my hesitancy. So, they sent me down to Houston to meet the current field rep, and he made arrangements to show me the town.

I flew to Houston, was picked up by the current field rep, and immediately went to lunch at a place I presume he surely thought would impress me. It was called Mickey Gilley's. It was famous in Houston and many other Texas towns. The rep wanted me to try some of their famous crawfish—something I'd never had before—as a good introduction to how *fun* it would be to live in Houston.

To make a long story short, I got sicker than a dog on those crawfish. I busted out in hives and spent the remainder of the day and night in my hotel room with diarrhea and burning, itching hives coloring my initial impressions of Houston. The current rep got to show me my hotel, and that was as far as he got. Needless to say, upon flying back to Peoria the next day and meeting with my bosses, I explained that I would have to turn down the assignment.

That triggered an almost frightening avalanche of activity. I thought I was going to be fired. Finally, in a personal one-on-one meeting with the *big boss*, I had to come clean. He began by saying, "Bill, we have a problem." He explained that I was hired to be mobile and declining this position was a huge negative for my employment prospects with the company. Finally, I told him the real reason for my declining the position. It wasn't Houston. It wasn't crawfish. It wasn't that the job wasn't a fit for me. It was primarily because I was trying to get my life right spiritually, and a move at this time was just not something I could do in complete peace. Amazingly, this wonderfully empathetic man and I discussed faith, repentance, my church, and my long-term goals and eventual willingness to get *back on track* with the mobility and relocation needs of the company. I was as honest as I could be, still being extremely nervous that I might be killing my career and potentially resulting in my termination from the Marketing Rep Program—if not the company as well.

Finally, the big boss leaned back in his chair and repeated his opening statement. "Well, Bill, we do have a problem." Long pregnant pause. I braced for the next words from his mouth. "But the problem is **not** Bill Mayo," he said. And I breathed a huge sigh of relief.

I thank God for that result. To be honest, Caterpillar was very accommodating. I was reassigned temporarily to Service Training and spent the next year getting my spiritual life together. (Well, I **thought** I was getting it together—more about that later.) For the moment, the pressure was off, and I was at peace. And that brings me to Howard.

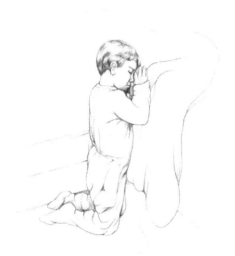

4

INTRODUCING HOWARD

Howard—the most important character in my story—is none other than God. God the Father, God the Son, and God the Holy Spirit. The Trinity, all three elements of God's divine nature, are part of my cancer journey.

I mean no disrespect to our Heavenly Father. As Christians will know, He has many names given in Scripture—Elohim (The Creator God), El Roi (The God who sees me), El Shaddai (Lord God Almighty), Yahweh Rophe (The God who heals), Yahweh Yireh (The Lord who provides), Yahweh-Raah (The Lord, my shepherd).

Howard is obviously a much less formal name and not a title at all. Much as Scripture tells us we may call upon our Heavenly Father as *Abba, Father*—a name that is as informal and relational as *Daddy*—my use of His name as *Howard* comes from a cute story I once heard so many years ago that I can't even attribute it to its rightful author. With apologies to that unknown writer, I'll re-tell his story here. The context is simply a child's innocent prayer of faith, overhead by his mother.

Momma stood in the bedroom doorway, quietly observing little Johnnie saying his nighttime prayers. She wore a proud yet warm smile for her sweet little boy. But while listening, her ears perked at his earnest pleas.

Johnnie prayed, "Dear Howard, please bless Mommy and Daddy. And Howard, bless my brother and sister, too. Oh, and Howard, bless my cousins, aunts, uncles, and everybody in the whole world. Thank you, Howard. Amen."

Momma stepped to Johnnie's bedside to tuck him in, and although touched by the sincerity of her child's heart-felt petitions, was more than mildly confused by the named recipient of his prayer. Curious, Momma asked, "Honey, uh, who's Howard?"

Johnnie replied, "Why, that's God, Mommy. You know that."

"God?" she asked.

"Yes, Mommy. That's what you and Daddy call Him, right?"

Still puzzled, Momma asked, "What do *we* call God, honey?"

Johnnie responded with unaffected innocence, "Well, you always pray 'Our Father, who art in heaven, *Howard* be Thy name'!"

It's a cute story and one that has stuck with me for many years. I've appropriated Johnnie's reference to *Howard* for my journey.

Simply stated, Howard is my God. And throughout this story, I hope to convey the very real presence He's had in my journey.

I hope none will take offense to my frequent reference to God as Howard. I mean no disrespect. It's as if I'm calling Him *Daddy,* and that is the spirit I intend. It's merely my elected style to make God more approachable and personal throughout this experience. He was very much with me, and His presence seemed like that of a wonderful personal friend—a *daddy*. If offense is the case for some reading this, I ask for your indulgence and your forgiveness.

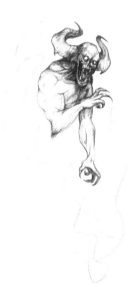

5

STANLEY – UP CLOSE AND PERSONAL

Now, I'd like to circle back to Dr. Jane Liu for a moment, as she was so instrumental in this whole adventure with Stanley and Houston. She is a cute, petite, dark-haired female with a ready smile and a compassionate heart. Both Gail and my eldest daughter, Erin, attended with me for our first meeting. Dr. Liu spent five or so minutes chatting about us. Nothing that would qualify as medical history—simply pleasant conversation just as one might have with any new acquaintance.

Finally, and perhaps a bit impatiently, I took my chance to segue into the point of the whole matter and asked, "So, what-taya' think about Stanley?"

She seemed puzzled and with a quizzical expression asked, "Who's Stanley?"

I then explained the derived name of my new resident tumor, and she accepted all of that with good humor. I knew I would like this lady doc. Erin took notes while Gail and I tried to focus on the words Dr. Liu spoke. I'm so glad Erin was our scribe, as it's a piece of notebook paper I still have today and am actually drawing from it for this narrative.

Dr. Liu stated that Stanley's formal name was more accurately Stage III Undifferentiated Pleomorphic Spindle Cell Sarcoma. I had no prior concept of what Stage III meant, but I instinctively thought that it was likely bad—one or two had to be better, I reasoned. Turns out, it wasn't as bad as it could be. Dr. Liu explained cancer staging and said that Stanley was a large, high-grade tumor with possible spread to lymph nodes but at this point had not yet metastasized. She said this particular type of cancer was rare, but what they did know about it was that the typical metastatic path was most commonly to the lungs and/or liver.

We asked for a breakdown of each term, and Dr. Liu smiled and said, "I am getting to that." She went on to explain that *undifferentiated* simply means the cells of the tumor look very abnormal and not much at all like normal cells. More specifically, she explained that the cancer cells of Stanley didn't resemble the body tissues in which they developed. Of course, this was not news to me because I had always assumed cancer cells must be some kind of weird morphed cells that went rogue and looked ghastly. Dr. Liu further explained what this meant for us was that they couldn't tell precisely where Stanley originated. That was more than a bit concerning because it implied that they really didn't know at this point if Stanley came from muscle cells or bone cells or any par-ticular organ—they just looked *very abnormal.*

Great, I thought, *Stanley could be hiding out* anywhere *in my body!*

The word *pleomorphic,* she continued, meant that Stanley's cells were growing in multiple shapes and sizes. I then asked about *spindle cells,* and she explained the obvious...Stanley's cells were spindle-shaped—or elongated ovals in the connective or fibrous tissue beneath the skin and around the bone, nerves, tendons, and blood vessels. Finally, *sarcoma* is the word for soft-tissue can-cers. Soft-tissue sarcomas can develop in blood vessels or in deep skin, muscle, fibrous or nerve tissues, and fat. Lord knows, I had plenty of fat to choose from! In particular, Stanley's cancer type usually occurs in the arms or legs and somewhat less often in the area behind the abdominal cavity. It can become quite large over a period of weeks or months, sometimes growing quite rap-idly. There are also slower growing sarcomas. I hoped Stanley was the more lethargic type. She said a rapidly-growing sarcoma would typically cause pain, and since to this point I'd had no pain symptoms at all, I was soothed, thinking Stanley might indeed be a sluggard.

Okay, so now that we knew a bit more about Stanley, it was clear I was not going to like him. Wanting to know how we were going to get along, I asked Dr. Liu, "So, what's the survival rate with this type of cancer?" Of course, I was being stoic, pseudo-brave, and asked the question like an interested party with mere intellec-tual curiosity—instead of the frightened guy sitting across from her.

Dr. Liu was facing the computer with her back to me as I asked this last question, and she pushed away from her keyboard, rolled her chair back, and turned around to face me. "Typically, fifty per-cent in five years."

Well, naturally, wanting to continue my stoic front and show no fear, I asked, "So, what is better—to try to treat this with chemo and radiation or do nothing and enjoy a good quality of life for as long as I have left?"

She smiled again and said with unfeigned confidence, "Oh, we're going to cure this!"

To her credit, and as I've previously mentioned, Dr. Liu explained that the local St. Francis Medical Center and Illinois Cancer Care Center would not provide the best assault versus Stanley. She asked if I would mind her referring me to her friend and colleague in Texas. "M.D. Anderson also has a dedicated sarcoma clinic," she added. For reasons previously expressed, while I wasn't particularly excited about it being in Houston, I affirmed to Dr. Liu that I was agreeable.

- 6 -

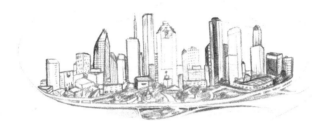

HOUSTON, WE
HAVE A PROBLEM

Most Americans will remember the calm declaration of astronaut John Swigert Jr. aboard the Apollo 13 mission. Following a major explosion on board the spacecraft, Swigert, without a hint of drama, coolly said, "Houston, we have a problem." Even though this familiar expression isn't exactly what Swigert said, it has nevertheless become a ubiquitous phrase of the American lexicon to report any kind of significant glitch. Well, Stanley, for us, was a significant glitch. Dr. Liu's referral to M.D. Anderson became the impetus for my statement, "Houston, we have a big problem." Someone later told me, "Don't tell God you have a big problem. Tell your problem you have a big God."

Of course, one of the dangers when you have only limited information about something attacking your body, like sarcoma, is that the temptation to begin reading everything you can find about it on the Internet is very high. I'm not prone to giving counsel, and this isn't an advice book, but I will bend my principle on this point. Be very careful turning to the Internet for reliable medical guidance. There's so much alarming and inaccurate bunk out there, it can be overwhelming at best and terribly frightening at the worst. It just encourages second-guessing of the medical team assembled to help you. It's far more profitable to spend more time reading about God than reading about cancer. I had to trust that in going to M.D. Anderson and their dedicated sarcoma clinic, I'd be in capable hands.

I did not heed my own advice, however. I personally yielded to the temptation to search the Internet, as I suspect most would. Looking back, while it's wise to be informed, I learned that one cannot squeeze a medical degree into a few hours of surfing the Net. Confusion reigns, and anxiety follows.

Following my frustrating and exhaustive search for definitive answers, Gail suggested it would be more prudent to reserve our questions for the medical team in Houston. We were blessed in that they were so approachable. We knew they were highly skilled; still, we prayed—along with our family and countless dear friends— that they would be guided by the Great Physician—*Howard.*

Believers talk about the peace that God can provide in the midst of a storm—*a peace that surpasses all understanding (Philippians 4:7).* Well, certainly, Gail and I felt the power of those many prayers. It gave us peace despite the fact that we were heading to Houston, sucked into the medical vortex to deal with that ugly word—*cancer.*

Our peace helped us approach each trip relatively calmly, and we also tried to include quite a few enjoyable things on the many trips we've had since that initial visit in August of 2012. We frequently drove because we both hate to fly. So, we'd take several days to drive and enjoy a little *vacation* en route. Shopping at secondhand stores. Detouring off the interstates to explore unique small towns. Finding the popular local café for a home-cooked meal. We had a lot of fun adventures en route.

We'd also typically tack on a visit to our friends Bob and Diane Cashen in Mobile, Alabama. And following the Alabama leg of our trips, we'd drive up Interstate 65 to visit our daughters and their families in Nashville. So, while each trip had its downside—tackling Stanley—we were blessed to also enjoy ourselves and refresh our spirits with visits to dear friends and family.

I'll admit that as much as I coveted those prayers that sustained us throughout this journey, I was very sheepish about asking for them. Everyone has their own struggles, and it felt almost intrusive to burden our friends with ours. But our friends were faithful, and we were humbled to know we were being prayed for. To be honest, it almost made me feel guilty to have so many praying for me specifically. It felt undeserved. I felt somewhat unworthy being the recipient of so much care and concern.

While I never admitted it to anyone except Gail, there was one other specific aspect to our first Houston trip that I was anxious about. I have to admit that it exposes one of my many regrets in life to retell it.

My mother died on April 16th, 2002. At the time, she and my sister and her family lived in Overland Park, Kansas. Cindy (my sister) and my mother were very close, but my brother and I lived far away. And sadly, we had let time and distance encumber our family relationships. I rarely spoke with my sister. My brother spoke with her even rarer still. So, when Mom died, we somewhat awkwardly came together for the *business end* of dying—funeral proceedings, a will, probate, disposition of assets, etc.

I've always called this the *administriva* of dying. It can be a lot of work to settle an estate. In the best of families, I've heard horror stories of conflict, disagreement, and contentious battles for one's fair share in such proceedings. Due to our physical distance from Kansas, my brother and I more than happily agreed with my sister that she fulfill the duties of executrix for Mom's modest estate. Though we weren't close, of course, we trusted her to manage things equitably, and, as I said, it was a modest estate anyway.

I don't want to be harsh here by smearing the memory of our sister, but my brother David and I were both quite disturbed by her handling of her executrix role. Suffice it to say that the division of assets greatly favored my sister, including her request for a rather significant executrix fee for her efforts. Both my brother and I were older and more well-established and didn't need the assets or material possessions. Thus, David and I conceded without objection just to avoid the nasty stereotypical feud of such situations.

I'm not justifying this but, admittedly, in an already-strained family dynamic, this episode exacerbated the division. And here is my regret...neither I nor my brother actually spoke with or visited our sister for many years following our mother's death. In my case, over nine years. Life was busy, we weren't close anyway, and, to my shame, I did not reach out to her at all. That is, until Howard intervened and directed my path on my journey with Stanley to Houston. Why then? Well, it wasn't because I thought I was going to die and needed to clean the slate—I didn't think that. So, what triggered my sudden willingness to meet up and reestablish relations with Cindy after over nine years?

Guess where my sister lived at that time? Texas! San Antonio to be precise, a mere three-hour drive from Houston. Howard put upon my heart that this would be the perfect time to reunite with my disenfranchised younger sibling. On our first visit to Houston, I discussed this burden with Gail, and she was "all in." She had frequently encouraged me to engage with Cindy through the years—calling our family spat *silly* and warning me that I'd regret it someday. She was right. So, on that first Houston trip, I did call my sister and asked if Gail and I could come visit. She agreed—and to my surprise, quite warmly so.

On the first free weekend we had, following a week filled with a countless array of medical appointments and tests, we drove the three hours to San Antonio. I was tentative and had a flood of conflicting emotions when we pulled into her driveway. But I mustered the proper frame of mind, exited our rental car, and found myself knocking on her door.

My sister, twelve years my junior, opened the door and gave me a warm hug. To say I was shocked would be a staggering understatement. She looked twenty years older than *me*! She looked disheveled and haggard. This was not the sister I last saw at Mom's funeral. She was considerably heavier, for one. But aren't we all? The shock came from her swollen eyes, her unkempt appearance, and most notably, her high-as-a-kite and slurred speech. She was clearly on some sort of medication that made her more than a little loopy. She talked like a recording played back at half-speed. Her ability to concentrate on one train of thought was clearly compromised. I was so stricken with shame that I had neglected this little sister of mine—the sister I had rocked to sleep as a little baby, the sister who adored me and was very close until I graduated high school and went away to college. I was choking back a lot of emotion. Gail observed the same thing in Cindy with equal alarm.

During the course of the next three hours, we had quite the conversation. I learned Cindy was a self-proclaimed reforming alcoholic. She admitted addiction to Xanax and some other anti-depressants. She stated that she formerly consumed a fifth of vodka a day and took lots of pills. All for pain, I was told—from a vague diagnosis of fibromyalgia. She said she'd cut down a lot on her alcohol consumption lately. *So much for recovering alcoholic,* I thought. And she stated that for a full six months, she was unable to get up from bed at all.

Ironically, my brother-in-law, Jerry, was in much the same shape, although much more lucid than Cindy was during the entirety of our visit. Still, his drug and alcohol abuse had caused the loss of many jobs in rapid succession, and he was currently unemployed at the time of our visit. They were deeply in debt and had no means to crawl out of their predicament, with few prospects for employment.

I can't relate how guilty I felt but also couldn't help discerning that Howard wanted me there. You can scoff if you like, but no other cancer would have likely taken me to Texas. Only the cancer sub-type I had would have reasonably required a referral to M.D. Anderson's renowned sarcoma clinic. So, there I was, with my very endangered sister who I'd ignored for nine-plus years, and she was clearly in need of my help. Before we left, I asked her about her faith. She and Jerry had at one time been active in church and were committed believers. Somehow, that had gone off the rails. She said they hadn't been to church for several years. I asked her if I could pray for her before we left. She asked me in that half-speed lilting tone, "Do you think something's wrong?"

I blurted out, "Cindy, are you kidding me? Of course, there's something wrong. You need help—both to get off drugs and alcohol and to re-engage with your faith and get your life together. And we will help you as we can."

She turned to Jerry and said, "See, Jerry, I told you Bill would see there was a problem!"

Again, I was shocked. How could I not see it? We had a prayer together, and I promised to stay close to help them get things squared away as best I could. Then, Gail and I departed with much to pray about on our three-hour drive back to Houston.

So, yes, Houston, we indeed had a problem. But the problem wasn't Stanley. He brought to me to Houston, and his presence turned out to be a part of the solution. Our frequent trips to Houston allowed me to regularly check in on Cindy to help resolve the real problem—to help restore my sister and help her find God again. Howard had a plan for that. His plan included a great deal of work on me as well. So, this is as good a time as any to segue to a deeper dive into *me.*

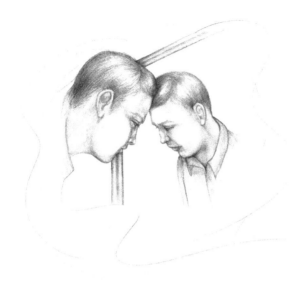

ME, UP CLOSE
AND PERSONAL

I n Chapter 3's brief introduction to *me*, I referenced my philosophy that we are all three people. Who we think we are. Who
we want others to think we are. And who we really are.

Well, to get up close and personal with the real me—who I
really am—I've had to strip away some of my own false perceptions. And for those who think they know me now, I'll have to strip
away some of those false perceptions I've fostered as well.

It is a humbling proposition to expose one's self in this manner, but to truly reflect Howard's and Stanley's impact upon *me*, I have to come clean, so-to-speak. It isn't perfected thinking—as if it ever could be—but it's raw and honest. And again, I'm being vulnerable to the point of perhaps foolishness—but it is cathartic, so I will proceed. First, some general orientation.

I am a local boy—a product of Illinois. I live today some twelve miles from where I was born. Although I've traveled the world, I am still very much homegrown. I did not grow up in a churched family. My mother was a devout believer, but my father was not—either by profession or by action. I was baptized as an infant, but we did not go to church as a family. I only remember my father attending church with us once. It was a Christmas Eve service, clearly a Christmas present for my mother.

Mom did endeavor to take my brother and me to church and Sunday school, but we boys weren't too keen on the idea. Cindy had not arrived in our family yet; she came later when I was in the sixth grade. So, it was just us two ornery boys. To reveal my strong-willed nature, I'll admit that in third grade, while supposedly attending Sunday school, a friend and I snuck out of the assembly room and walked to a local hospital just a few blocks away. We quite boldly walked through the ward hallways, looking for donuts to steal. We found some in the maternity ward! My mom never knew.

I did attend confirmation classes in the Lutheran church and was confirmed in eighth grade. While that may have satisfied some desire of my mother's, for me, it was merely a bothersome chore. It meant nothing to me and only confirmed my passage through some obligatory milestone.

I moved around a lot during my school years. I attended six different grade schools and two different high schools. This certainly had an impact upon me and how I engaged my world but not as much impact as my strained family situation.

I've teased for years that my father used to always say, "Everyone's good for something—even if it's being a bad example." He didn't necessarily direct this to me, specifically, but I heard it. I heard it a lot. Enough that it's seared into my memory. One thing I do remember him saying to me, specifically, on many occasions when he'd arrive home from work, was this…

"You been good today?"

Naturally, and quite automatically, I'd reply, "Yes, Dad."

He'd then follow up with his favorite set-up line. "Did you get paid for being good?"

"Nope," I'd respond.

And then he'd deliver his all-too-familiar punchline: "Then you're good for nothing!"

He always got a big chuckle from that exchange. To this day, I'm not quite sure how I felt about it then or feel about it now. I only know that it was unforgettable, and there's good reason for my uncertainty about its emotional impact.

When I was twelve years old, I had one of those grueling early morning paper routes. Rain or shine or freezing weather, just like the U.S. Post Office, I delivered. I and dozens of other young paperboys in town would rise early, get our papers, load them in our bicycle baskets, and head out to deliver the news of the day.

One early winter morning, I woke up to the sounds of my mother and father arguing in the kitchen. Arguing wasn't necessarily a new thing in our family; my brother and I were exposed to a lot of it. My bedroom was a small room just off the kitchen. I couldn't help but overhear anything going on in there. The gist of their arguing was about us boys again— my brother David and me. This spat dug a little deeper than most because it was mostly about me. I remember hearing my dad yelling, "Billy's a baby. He's always been a baby. He'll always be a baby! David's a man. And Billy's not my son!"

I was stunned. Did I just hear that? I heard my mom exclaim, "Of course, he's your son!"

After that, the argument spilled from the kitchen into their bedroom, and while I could still hear their raised yet muffled voices, I could not distinguish what was being said. Just as well...I'd heard enough to last a lifetime. And it almost did.

Being wide awake, I busied myself with getting dressed. I donned my winter coat, scarf, and gloves; went to the garage; got on my bike; and headed out—saying goodbye to no one. I went to my newspaper pick-up spot, gathered my papers, and delivered my route—all the while with his words, "He's not my son," echoing a cutting refrain in my brain.

I tell that story and the ones that follow about my father's relationship with me—**not** to elicit sympathy nor compassion but because it shaped my life and image of self, as well as my *intended projection* of self tremendously, well into my adult years.

Before going on, I want to emphatically proclaim that I loved my father then. And I love him now. I've forgiven him his shortcomings because like all of us, he had his baggage. He had a difficult life, and what he experienced would be traumatic for anyone. It no doubt scarred him deeply. I do not want to minimize what he did and didn't do nor vilify him in a way that marks him as unforgiveable. He was my dad. I love him and pray that he found his peace and reconciliation with our Heavenly Father.

The impact of his denial of my relationship to him was indeed significant. It wasn't so much that I believed I was "good for nothing"—even though I never heard my dad use that exchange even once with my brother. It wasn't that I was called a baby—because in fact, I was a sensitive little kid, and I'm sure to a *man's man* like my father, I seemed a bit wimpy. What stung and continued to sting well into adulthood was the overriding sense of rejection I felt. I was not my father's son. Which meant, of course, that he did not love me as a son.

By the time I came home from my paper route, Dad had already left for work. I was glad because I had those big *Baby Billy* tears welling in my eyes. Mom noticed at once and asked what was the matter. I broke down and confessed I had heard their argument.

With tears and trembling lips, I asked, "Is Dad my father?"

Mom came across the kitchen to me and held me close. We moved to the kitchen table, and she sat me down, sitting across from me. She told me that I was absolutely my father's son. Then she explained that Dad thought I was an illegitimate offspring of an affair he had accused her of having. I didn't even really know what an *affair* was until she told me, but I knew the important part of the accusation. He did not claim me as his.

My mom tried to reassure me. She said just to look to the family resemblance—it was undeniable. I knew my mother was a moral Christian woman. I didn't need her to deny an affair to know it wasn't true. I learned that my father thought one of his restaurant vendors—a Bunn Coffee supplier—was, in fact, sweet on my mother. But it wasn't reciprocated. Perhaps this explains why I still don't like coffee today!

In subsequent talks with my mother over the years, this unfortunately was a recurring conversation. I had a lot of difficulty getting over that supreme sense of rejection. As a result, I spent the majority of my life attempting to gain my father's and others' approval. That quest for his approval extended into basically every arena of my life. I sought approval from any and everyone—just because I needed it so acutely.

I suppose that need wasn't all bad, however. If there was a silver lining to my feelings of rejection, it was that it created an intense drive within to prove I was "good for something"— and that I was worthy of acceptance and love. I suppose I could have chosen to go into the darkness of retreat, to shrink away or to quit, but I didn't do that. Instead, I was determined to earn approval through accomplishment.

I had a tremendous need to excel, to earn acceptance, to earn admiration, and to earn love. Therefore, I worked hard at it. I excelled at school. I was good in sports. I strived for popularity and acceptance in virtually any and every social setting. I graduated with high standing and received merit scholarships and academic accolades from high school. I received a Congressional appointment to the U.S. Naval Academy, which I attended—again, to please my very pro-military dad.

Yet I never heard my father say he was proud of me. Not once. I never felt his acceptance, while seeing it lavished on my brother. I never **earned** the love I craved, despite my achievements. I certainly did not understand that love and acceptance for achievement were not what I actually craved. I craved love and acceptance just for being.

To be fair, my father did express his love for me one time. I was twenty-five years old and a lieutenant in the United States Navy. I was executive officer of a U.S. Navy warship. That particular day, my dad was aboard the ship on which I was stationed. It was Family Day Open House hosted by my commanding officer. Standing on the bridge of the ship, after I gave my father the nickel tour of the entire vessel, he did tell me he loved me. It was a bit of an awkward moment. He moved to hug me, and I stiffened. I don't even remember what I said in reply.

At least he had said it. He loved me. At that point in time, however, the echoes of "He's not my son" were louder than the one "I love you" he expressed. So, I didn't believe it. I couldn't believe it. I'd lived a quarter of a century striving and seeking his approval. Hearing this expression just felt empty, forced. Since that early morning revelation so many years prior, I had become addicted to approval from all but, internally, never felt I had it. His expression did not erase that feeling. I could achieve many things but achieving a sense of love and acceptance was elusive. No matter what I achieved or how I excelled, I not only didn't believe I had approval or love, I didn't believe it was even attainable.

My striving for approval had many, many dark sides, too. It led to bad choices—in relationships, in unseemly activities, and in my spiritual life as well. It led to a perverted neediness and narcissism. If no one loved me, or worse, no one *could* love me, I reasoned, then I would simply put myself first. I would love me. And it became all about me.

So that's who I really was—a self-centered, narcissistic individual who needed approval from others, but would never allow anyone close enough to hurt or reject me. Of course, that's **not** what I wanted others to think I was. I wanted them to see something quite different.

I put forth an image of a strong-willed, determined, focused, and competitive person— strong physically, mentally, and emotionally, such that I could tackle any challenge and plow through it to a successful end. I projected confidence. I projected an image of a winner. No challenge was going to defeat me. I was as determined as one could be to get to the top of the mountain—whatever that mountain might be. I pretended to be totally self-sufficient. I didn't need anybody at the time, even though in reality, I needed everyone to love me. I thought I could muscle through life. Oh, I still had my tender side, but it was hidden from most.

The image I wanted others to see became my singular focus— to project the *me* that I thought would most likely gain approval. My quest for approval was my drug. And I needed a continual fix.

Truth be told, this worked for me. I became a standout academically and in the sports arena. I was popular. People saw what I wanted them to see. My image was also my defense mechanism. If no one could get past that image to get close to me, no one could hurt me. No one could reject me. Sometimes it led to people reading me as aloof or arrogant or, at best, just stand-offish or shy. That I could handle. Rejection, I couldn't.

For anyone who knows me today, this may be perceived as a concocted story. One written to elicit obligatory affirmations of how *great* I am or to solicit vehement denials that the above admissions of my obvious flaws couldn't be true. Trust me. The reality is, they are true. It's taken a lot of Howard's working on me—sanctifying me over a long course of time—to allow me to mentally process through it and, more importantly, to change. Stanley had a big impact on that.

When Stanley entered my life, I had to come to a new realization. I was forced to realize that I was no longer that *tough guy*. I was vulnerable. I was dependent upon others. I couldn't muscle through Stanley. I needed others. And I needed Howard.

At M.D. Anderson, I faced countless days subjected to whatever medical processes, tests, pokes and sticks, and procedures that were prescribed. I was not in control. I feared this could be my new normal for an extended period of time—months, maybe years. Howard knew this would ultimately and systematically strip me of my physical, emotional, mental, social, and even perhaps intellectual toughness that I'd come to define as *me*.

I am ashamed to reveal this next episode in my life but being fully transparent requires that I do so. I had supposedly accepted Christ when I was sixteen years old. Truth be told, it was an emotional experience where I got caught up in the moment and came forward to accept Christ at one of those popular high school youth events. Oh, I think it changed me for a month or two, but in no time, I was back to the tough-minded, hard-headed, and rebellious Bill I'd been prior to that. Not until my late twenties, after the Navy and just beginning my career at Caterpillar, did I decide to repent and become a member of my local church and begin living a Christian life. There must have been some lingering sense that I needed a Savior after that experience at sixteen.

At twenty-eight, I made a formal testimony, was baptized again, and professed my belief, knowing even as I stood in the baptismal waters that I both believed and didn't believe. I am mortified to admit it, but it's true. I earnestly believed. And I earnestly had doubts. I was so unstable I could experience a complete switch-eroo from one position to the other in the same day. True belief requires surrender, and I wasn't quite willing to do that—to give up the construct of *me* that I had created.

I had held such doubts intellectually for a long time. You can chalk it up to so-called Christians disappointing me or what I viewed as man-made religion disappointing me. Either way, I still had my doubts, similar to what I wrote about in my senior year of high school. My final term paper for English Composition was entitled *Death May Be Man's Greatest Reward*. In it, I quoted several philosophers I was into at the time (who were categorically **not** Christian). They definitely influenced my thinking, so much so that I struggled with faith long after I had purposed in my mind to change my life.

My brother no doubt also greatly influenced this line of thinking. He was not a believer. Frankly, I didn't need a lot of encouragement to question. I stubbornly held onto these doubts from my earlier days—no doubt impacted by my view that I was unlovable—even by a God who *is love.*

David and I would often challenge each other to read a passage from the Bible and come prepared to debate it. Me from the position of faith, supposedly, and he from the position of the agnostic. One time, we discussed John 1:1-13—a very familiar passage, I'm sure. "In the beginning was the Word, and the Word was with God, and the Word was God...et cetera, et cetera."

This debate really shook my already wobbly standing in faith. We discussed these verses at length. It was actually I who suggested that these verses could possibly prove that the Christian faith was man's creation. Using these verses, I reasoned that what controls man is his thoughts. And if the beginning was just *the Word*—essentially the manifestation of man's thoughts— then with merely a bit of convoluted logic, one possible interpretation of the reading could be that man *invented* God. He was merely a creation of man's thoughts, plainly stated right in the Bible. From an intellectual and philosophical perspective, this appealed to me. It made sense. And it was easier than blind faith, to be frank.

Together, we paraphrased the verses, suggesting that "In the beginning, man had a thought. A thought that he made into a god. And he gave it flesh and blood and made up a whole story about him." It wasn't a huge stretch to then postulate that man's **mind** was actually **the** god.

To me today, this is a shameful episode of backsliding! But it happened, and as I said, it shook me and my confidence in faith big time. My assurance in Howard was tentative. Clearly, my feet were not on the *Rock* but on some very shifting sands.

Not long thereafter, I was reading in the book of 2 Peter and encountered 2 Peter 1:16: "For we have not followed cunningly devised fables, but were eyewitnesses to His majesty." I discussed this discovery with David. He firmly held his position, but I couldn't reconcile the two readings. One section seemed to say, "Man made it all up with his thoughts." The other seemed to say, "Hey, man, you can't make this stuff up. It isn't some clever tale. We were **there**!" Eyewitnesses! Eyewitnesses who in many cases lost their lives professing belief in Jesus Christ as Savior. It was a powerful argument.

Thankfully, the Lord got me out of my own **head** and began to work on my heart. I am humiliated by this episode in my life, but I came by it honestly. Being unchurched as a kid, not having a harmonious Christian home, and not observing each family role model live out their faith from day to day, along with my own reading of babbling atheist philosophy, all contributed to my distorted view of faith, of God.

It's amazing and humbling to me now, in addition to being very embarrassing, to realize God loved me enough to pull me through all that stuff, all that erroneous thinking. Howard could have (and should have) spewed me out of **His** mouth. Instead, He warmly embraced me and guided me to the light. He brought a godly woman into my life, Gail, to be my wife. She patiently (but with some significant consternation, I'm certain), immeasurably aided in my eventual transformation. Today, I realize that the closer we are to the light, the smaller the shadow becomes. The farther from the light we are, the longer the shadow becomes. I thank Howard that He delivered me from the shadows and brought me closer to Him—closer to the light.

I love reading John 1 today. With full confidence, I know that it means Jesus was with God and *was* God from the beginning— before the world was created. I cannot read it today without reflecting upon how much of an idiot I was and how much I hurt and offended Howard.

Getting through that type of flimsy intellectual mindset was a long journey. Howard had freed me from some of that philo- sophical crap, but believing and living are miles apart. And I still did not completely live as if I needed Him. In my spiritual life, I was still the *me* who tried to muscle it. Submission was not my strong suit. When I joined Caterpillar and claimed I was trying to get my spiritual life in order, that was true. But while I repented of my prior sins, I was still that tough-minded, self-sufficient, and approval-seeking kid. I lived my spiritual life as I lived my entire life—aloof from needing anyone, including Howard.

This version of *me* created a lot of tension in my life and, to my shame, caused much tension in my family and marriage. From the outside, things looked good, sounded good, and smelled good— but living as I lived, so selfishly, was anything but good. Not good for me or good for others. I had set my sails on a course that refused to truly need anyone. I went to church. I worshipped— sort of. I served in various church positions. I even taught Sunday school. I had a relationship with Howard, but it was more like second cousins. I'd see Him once in a while, but by and large, He wasn't a big part of my daily life. He was my Sunday life, and I was merely going through the motions.

On more than one Sunday morning, I would dress in my suit, walk my kids to church, go through the kitchen to see a few folks (more honestly to be *seen* by a few folks), and then I would walk through the lobby, down the back hall, and out the back door. I'd slip into a nearby alleyway and walk home—off the main street, so as to not be seen—and would go home to watch football. My wife would be asked, "Where's Bill?" And, of course, she'd reply, "Oh, he's here somewhere." That was the beauty of a large congregation—I would be seen by a few to corroborate and confirm my attendance, but I was missed by many, attributable to the big crowd of church-goers. This was all, again, part of the meticulous image I wanted and needed to project of being a good, God-fearing man. All the while, I ignored the damage in my wake—damage to my spiritual life and damage to others who cared for me.

Stanley and Howard challenged all of that. Both caused me to confront the reality that I *had* no toughness—no mental toughness, no physical toughness, no emotional toughness—and certainly challenged my spiritual aloofness. All I had was *need*. And that dependency was difficult to swallow.

While I knew the Bible declared, "His strength is perfected in **my** weakness," (2 Corinthians 12:9) I was one who had no intention of admitting weakness. Lying in a hospital bed with multiple tubes running into my body, spilling nasty chemotherapy drugs into my system, made me come to the realization that I was now face-to-face with the end of *me* as I'd come to define myself. Sixty-plus years of my carefully crafted lie were at risk. I wasn't that hardened guy anymore. I couldn't be. In other words, the very way I'd defined myself as a person on this earth was **entirely** fleeting and totally false.

It was sobering. In a very real sense—not to be overly dramatic here—a part of the *me* I'd always thought I was and who I'd projected myself to be *was* dying. Not in a biological sense, of course, but in an emotional and spiritual sense. I remember wondering, "Is this what dying to self really means?" I'd always thought it meant dying to my own desires, but perhaps—at least in my case—it meant dying to the artificial construct I had made of my life.

Over the course of whatever time I had left, I concluded that my former image of self had to yield to a new reality of a hobbled, weaker individual. Someone who must admit he *did* indeed need others. And someone who needed love and acceptance just as I was—a flawed and damaged person—and *not* as the accomplished person I tried to project. I needed to strip away the façade and become real, become vulnerable, and become submissive to a power much greater than me.

I firmly believe that Howard directed Stanley into my life experience as my *second cancer*. I now realize my first cancer was the cancer of self. The old Bill needed to yield to a new reality of being a Bill who wasn't **at all** whom I'd tried to project to others.

As frightening as that realization was, however, Howard presented it as more of an opportunity. Instead of focusing on achievement and the need for approval of others, instead of thinking my achievements defined me, instead of focusing on myself, and instead of focusing on a *To Do* list of accomplishment, I could now focus on a *To Be* list. A list of qualities and attributes I desired to *be*—genuine, loving, accepting, happy, a good husband, and a good father but, most importantly, a *true* follower of Jesus Christ.

A believer who didn't merely profess it but one who lived it, believing from the very core of his being. Ironically, the God I felt I didn't need was actually the Father I could have always had. He made me. He'd directed my path to this point. And despite the flawed sinner that I was, through His Son Christ Jesus, He loved me. He forgave me. I'd finally found acceptance, approval, and the love that I craved—loved as a *son* by a Father who wholeheartedly claimed me as His. It was liberation!

And that compels me to take a closer look at Howard and His orchestration of my journey.

- 8 -

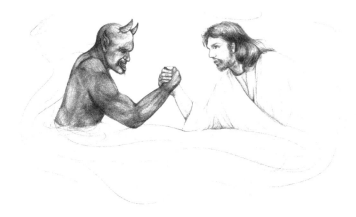

HOWARD, UP CLOSE
AND PERSONAL

I approach this chapter with trepidation. I know I will not adequately convey Howard's impact throughout this journey. It's intimidating, but I must try.

As I said, I firmly believe Howard directed Stanley into my life. I say "directed" without casual intent. Stanley wasn't just something Howard *allowed*. I know there is a common affirmation among believers that God won't give you anything more than you can handle. I don't feel I handled anything. I was just along for the ride. Howard knew I needed Stanley. It wasn't something He

47

permitted to occur but something He provided as a gift. Sounds crazy—cancer as a gift—but in my case, I feel as if Stanley was indeed gifted to me. I needed Stanley for a few reasons—to reconcile with my sister, to finally nudge David toward faith, to force me to confront the artificial construct I had made of my life, and also, to enable me to experience that indeed, His strength is made perfect in my weakness.

In the battle of Stanley versus me, Stanley versus the medical world, and Stanley versus Howard, I was a spectator and not in control. People would tell me, "You're tough; you'll fight this." In reality, it was not my battle to fight. It was Howard's. And I believed that with Howard at the helm of this voyage, I would win either way.

Howard reminded me that you always find what you're looking for. For example, when I was young and wanted a Volkswagen, all I saw on the highway were VW Bugs. Similarly, when Gail was pregnant with each of our five children, all I saw were pregnant women. You see what you want to see. This is also true when looking for Howard. When you look for Him, you'll see Him everywhere. In big moments, sure—but more often, in the little moments of life, which Gail and I have come to term *Howard Moments*.

Stanley provided more than a few opportunities to witness those Howard Moments. Some were small, and one could argue coincidental, but I don't believe they were chance. Some were huge, and I suspect you'll agree were undeniable. All were impactful to me. I will confess that it was those small moments that served to let me know He was directing my path, that He was in charge. In countless ways, those were the most encouraging.

Prior to actual hospitalization, Howard directed many special people into my life. I met a great number of cancer survivors—some I knew and some new to me. The brotherhood of cancer does something to people. In many ways, it strips away self-reliance and encourages them to share their experiences. Some people I had known surprised me with their cancer stories. I had no idea they had walked that road. Both groups willingly shared their stories and provided great encouragement. These encounters were not chance meetings. Without my realizing it, Howard was prepping me for the journey ahead.

People have often commented about my ability to face Stanley with a genuine sense of humor. Gail once asked me, "Are you really doing as well as you seem? Or are you faking it?" I don't fault her for her doubts. She'd seen me through many years where I'd portrayed that glass-half-empty persona I'd perfected. It would be understandably difficult for her to reconcile the positivity I'd displayed throughout Stanley's story with the struggling spirit I'd so often revealed in earlier years. But trust me, I don't have sufficient energy to maintain such a charade for over eight years!

Of course, I did experience significant lows. It would be disingenuous to puff myself up by projecting a false sense of confidence in the face of such daunting challenges. I wrestled with my demons of doubt and anxiety at times. I did have moments of fatigue and defeat. But I can also state, without a hint of contrived perspective, that through it all, Howard was with me. He enveloped me in a peaceful shroud, nurturing me through the difficulties, while also impressing upon me that I had a responsibility to give Him the glory. I knew my family was watching and perhaps so were others. I had an opportunity to display grace that couldn't emanate from within myself without Him putting it there. So, yes, Howard enabled me to maintain a humorous perspective on my struggles.

In those dark moments, how did I feel? How did I *feel* when faced with the relentless onslaught of chemo drugs? Or when I reeled from the two-time recurrence of Stanley? How did I feel when facing the bizarre prospect of losing my leg and my independence?

I felt like anyone would feel—overwhelmed. Despite those natural feelings of despair, each episode of trial was attended by a peace that only Howard could provide. I felt as if Howard was right there alongside me. I felt the encouragement of His Word in Isaiah 63:9: "In all their affliction He was afflicted, and the angel of His presence saved them: in His love and in His pity, He redeemed them; and He bare them, and carried them all the days of old."

Plus, admittedly, it's a lot easier to sustain a sense of humor when you're not doing the work! I was told that attitude definitely helps in healing. I wholeheartedly agree. I had a divine model for that sense of humor as well, as Howard displayed His awesome sparkle in many subtle ways.

For example, when I first met my M.D. Anderson oncologist, Dr. Neeta Somaiah, I was impressed with her. She was friendly, engaging, and clearly was a physician with great humanity and compassion. After the obligatory period of getting acquainted, I again did my Stanley introduction.

"So, tell us how we're gonna' tackle Stanley," I blurted.

Gail, likely embarrassed at my silly approach, explained that Stanley was the name given to my tumor by my grandkids. Dr. Somaiah smiled. She accepted Stanley's name as a clinical fact—even wrote it down.

She said, "We have a common enemy then—Stanley. Good to know!" To her credit, she continually referred to Stanley throughout our many encounters.

I believe Howard was assembling the perfect team for the battle versus Stanley.

Her referral to my oncological surgeon, a Puerto Rican-born physician named Dr. Keila Torres, permitted another chance to introduce Stanley to my expanding medical team. I informed her of the demon she'd be fighting—namely, Stanley—and she looked quizzically at me, as if I was one very odd duck.

Then she simply said, "Who's Stanley?" I let her in on the familial name given to my tumor, and she simply said, "Sorry for my confusion. My dog's name is Stanley!" She, too, throughout our many appointments always referred to Stanley with an impish grin.

I found out later that Dr. Torres is the author of *Teaching Your Dog and You*. Her book is based on her love of training dogs and her experiences with her three loving Labrador retrievers—Stanley, Albert, and Emma. She writes of her experience using positive reinforcement and how this method of training results in reliable, obedient behavior in pets. I hoped she would find *my* Stanley equally as obedient! Interestingly, Dr. Torres chose to pursue sarcoma research and surgery after losing a loved one to this very disease. She also told me that sarcoma is the most common form of cancer in our furry best friends. So clearly, Howard had assembled a team fully invested in defeating my nemesis.

Following the first tumor resection, Dr. Torres asked if I would be willing to sign a release permitting the hospital to send Stanley to pathology and then on to the research laboratory, where a research physician would map Stanley's genome. I was happy to oblige. In perfect Howard-scripted irony, the research doc's name was Stanley—Dr. Stanley Hamilton! Coincidence? Or just Howard having some sport? I believe the latter, and it makes me smile.

During the initial meeting with Dr. Somaiah, she explained we'd be tackling Stanley with eight cycles of chemotherapy and about four weeks of radiation. Following that, there would be surgery with Dr. Torres to remove Stanley—her exact words, by the way. As I've explained, I was blessed to have the twenty-eight days of chemo in my hometown. That was the good news. The bad news was the intensity of the chemo drugs prescribed. It wasn't lost on me that this was Howard's battle to wage, as the primary chemo drug prescribed was commonly referred to as *The Red Devil*. The Red Devil is, of course, a red liquid, looking quite ominous just dangling there beside me.

This is an apropos moment to discuss the impact of my chemo, as this was a major portion of the initial battle waged with Stanley. While these symptoms did not all occur at the same time, they occurred with significant regularity throughout the course of my treatments and cause me to undeniably declare that chemo is worse than the disease.

On the list of side effects that frequently occur in five to sixty percent of patients using the Red Devil was a symptom broadly labeled as *visual disturbances*. That label didn't even begin to cut it for me. For one, a very important adjective was omitted— *terrifying* visual disturbances—full-blown hallucinations during both waking hours or dreams. These exacerbated the nausea and severe headaches I was experiencing from the drugs, as well. The visions were dark in both tone and nature—evil, in a word. It was a metaphorical depiction of a bona fide spiritual battle.

The only thing I can comparatively offer to give you some sense of the nature and character of the images is the word *gargoyle-esque*. The images were dynamic—not like touring an art gallery but more as if engaging in combat or with me running fearfully from these grotesque and demon-like images. They tore at my clothes and skin and attempted to drag me into a dark pit. In the small confines of my hospital room, with IV poles supporting a rectangular device with blinking lights and buzzers and bags of various drugs emptying into my body, there was no escape.

The demons literally seemed intent on attacking and chipping away at my very sanity. The images were always black and white, except on the fourth day of the first week of chemo, when I visualized myself awake with a shiny, white three-headed cat sporting a red bow, sitting in my lap. It was smoking one of those long filter cigarettes with ribbons of grey smoke pirouetting above it. I have no idea what this symbolized, but while a bit humorous, it was also very disturbing. Was it a metaphor for Caterpillar attacking me? Or just some weird cat wearing the color of the Red Devil? I wasn't sure, but I was sure of one thing. Anxiety.

I became afraid to go to sleep. The attacks disturbed my daily rest as well, driving me to become mentally foggy while awake. I became increasingly fearful and off-balance. The hallucinations were uncontrollable, continual, and very destabilizing. Attendant with those hallucinations was a heightened sense of frustration— even anger—that I could do nothing to rid myself of them or to regain some semblance of mental control.

There were other aspects of chemo that were nasty, too. I learned one aspect was a symptom labeled *chemo brain*. I had difficulty speaking coherently to Gail or my kids. I had trouble forming (or remembering) thoughts, selecting the right word, or even keeping a string of cogent thought together without long, awkward moments of silence.

I remember feeling as if the real-time world around me was not my world. I felt as if it moved around me, and I was about five to ten seconds behind it. In terms of my ability to process move-ment, conversation, and articulate speech, I was dull and woozy. I was undermined and frustrated—Gail would add *angry*—at my inability to control my thoughts.

Chemo put me in a very dark, uncontrolled, and disturbing place. My emotions were on high alert as well. Tears were not infrequent. After the second full week of chemo, I broke down to my daughter Erin, admitting, "I'd rather have my leg cut off than go through Round 3!" How prophetic that turned out to be some eight years later.

There were other chemo side effects as well. There was minor tightening of the chest but not truly shortness of breath. Mouth dryness and sores, but these were relatively easy to treat with a special mouthwash. Tongue sores were a bit more bothersome. I also experienced moderate-to-nasty acid reflux and also itchy red welts and, oftentimes, insomnia.

If it's not yet clear, I thought chemo sucked big time. A nurse told me, "Chemo is administered in hopes that it kills the cancer before it kills you!" Amen! But still, I tried to remember Exodus 14:14: "The LORD shall fight for you, and ye shall hold your peace."

There were hefty Howard moments as well. After four cycles of that nasty chemo, I was depleted, with very little, if any, emotional or physical margin remaining. I was at my limit. I was sick, vomiting, frequently falling, and also neutropenic—meaning very susceptible to infection. I'd had two blood transfusions and was extremely weak. I had to wear one of those surgical masks, especially in the airports when we'd make our routine follow-up visits to Houston after each cycle. Following the fourth cycle, I again broke down into tears. I told Gail I could **not** endure the four additional cycles remaining.

My visit with Dr. Somaiah after that fourth cycle began with her physician's assistant doing a routine exam and prepping me for the doctor. I told her I could **not** take another cycle of chemo. She simply gave me the party line.

"Well, unfortunately, you have to take eight cycles." Adding cheerfully, "Only four more to go!"

If I could have reached her, I'd have punched her. Instead, after she left the exam room, I began to whimper again. Gail tried to comfort me, but without effect. I simply did not know how I could face four more weeks under the Red Devil's assault. Howard knew this, too.

Dr. Somaiah entered the room with a knock, and we said hello. She gave me a hug. My first words to her were, "If you tell me I have to take four more cycles of the Red Devil, I give up."

She smiled and said, to my complete surprise (but not Howard's), "Well then, I have good news for you. I'm stopping the chemo and shifting to the radiation protocol." I was shocked, relieved, and immediately, but silently, thanked Howard.

She explained that the chemo was having negligible effect on Stanley's size. As difficult as the chemo was with such minimal impact, it was time to move on to protocol number two...radiation. She referred me to the radiation clinic for the prescribed twenty-five days of radiation. We stayed in a local hotel during those weeks, but every morning at 6:30 am, we would drive to the radiation clinic for a mere two minutes of treatment. On my way in each morning, I noticed something and smiled. Every day we'd pass through an immense automatic glass door, and atop the door in big bold letters was the word *STANLEY*! Of course, I realize that Stanley is a popular manufacturer of such doors, but what were the odds? Howard gave me continual and humorous signals that He was directing the journey, and that I should just relax, hang on, and roll with it.

Further evidence of Howard's presence...as mentioned, my chemo treatments were administered locally at OSF Healthcare System in my hometown of Peoria, Illinois. Each treatment was a week long—twenty-four hours a day in the hospital. This would be followed by two weeks off and then back again. In the two-week respite between sessions, after three or four days, I would begin to feel a bit better. That made it all the more difficult to get my head around going back into the hospital every fourth week, knowing I was just going to feel sick and miserable again. Howard invoked His plan.

I credit Him with sending many visitors to keep my spirits up as I endured those tortuous weeks. Why credit Howard with this simple matter? It takes a good deal of effort and commitment to visit someone in a hospital—it's a deliberate act and often not convenient. I myself know I never enjoyed it when it was my turn to visit someone hospitalized. I remember how He put that burden on my heart that it was something I needed to do, not for myself but for the person laid up. Howard no doubt impressed upon many that a visit to the hospital might be a good thing for their friend

Bill. I'm grateful He moved in their hearts and they gave of their time to make my stays more tolerable.

A goodly number did come to visit. One was a dear friend from Bradley University by the name of Dr. Rob Prescott. Rob is chair of the English department at Bradley and was my mentor while pursuing my master's degree. Rob is one of the most positive, upbeat people I know. When he came in, he immediately sensed I was in distress. I had lost all my hair by this time, of course; I was puking and weak; my skin was a hideous pale grey. I'm sure I looked like death warmed over. Rob and I chatted for a while, and I shared the frightening hallucinations I'd been experiencing. Rob, a believer, looked around and noticed that although I was in a Catholic-affiliated hospital, there was no cross hanging in my room. There were **always** crosses in the patient rooms at Saint Francis hospital facilities, and the absence in my room to Rob was a glaring deficiency. He immediately went to maintenance, and within five minutes, there was a maintenance employee tacking a crucifix on my wall. One I could look at every day, directly across from my hospital bed.

I shared one specific hallucination from the night before with Rob. I woke in the middle of the night. The clock on the wall facing me was shrinking and expanding while the hands twisted grotesquely, spinning around the dial. It went on for a minute or more. I was sweating and panicking and considerably freaked out. That evening, I expressed that same new hallucination to the night nurse. She faithfully reported my complaint to the attending physician as well. He prescribed vitamin B-6 shots.

The next morning, less than twenty-four hours after Rob had placed the cross, I did not experience those disturbing visions again. I texted Rob and told him the Red Devil had been held at bay the previous evening. The attending doc said, "I'm glad the B-6 worked." Rob texted back saying, "We both know it was the cross!"

One more good friend and colleague, Ali Bahaj, dropped by. We'd talked by phone before, so he knew I was feeling more than a bit stripped of my masculinity by losing my hair. He showed up with, of all things, an Elvis wig. I share a birthday with Elvis, and this was just the ticket. I donned the wig, looking ridiculous with the stark black hair framing pale grey skin. We had a few laughs, and then Ali told me not to worry because an article in the *Atlantic Journal* had recently reported that shaved-head men appear taller (by one whole inch) and stronger (by thirteen percent) than normal-haired men. I'm not sure who comprised the polling audience, but both Ali and I had a good chuckle, and clearly Howard had a good sense of comedic timing as well!

Chemo made all food taste metallic. Nothing tasted good, which affected my appetite and desire to eat. Just the smell of those too often re-used hospital food plate covers was enough to elicit a retching feeling in my stomach. Howard sent my brother to see me with the solution. Black licorice! It tasted great and cleansed that metallic taste from my mouth. Regular food still tasted metallic, but my brother kept me in a steady supply of licorice—on the QT, of course! Gail would be appalled if she knew I was eating sugar since she always warned me that cancer loved sugar. On that point, Stanley and I were in complete agreement.

I would be remiss if I didn't mention the impact of prayer throughout this journey. We were blessed to have a great number of friends and family praying for us both throughout this long passage. And praying for the caregiver, Gail, was just as important, if not more so, than prayers for me. As mentioned, we come from a large, loving church. A church that, when bad news befalls someone, the jungle drums beat at once, both swiftly and reliably throughout the entire congregation. Soon cards and letters, phone calls, and texts poured in—all assuring us of a commitment to pray for us.

The phrase, "I'll pray for you," rolls easily off the tongue. Too easily. I've said it myself countless times after someone shared a problem with me. Trouble is, while my intentions may have been good, more often than not, I likely didn't remember to pray at all. My own selfish interests or priorities overcrowded the best of my intentions. In so many instances, no prayers went forth. Howard revealed how important it is to act upon that statement and not merely offer it as an empty expression of empathy.

Gail and I actually felt the prayers—*viscerally*. We *knew* we were being lifted up in prayer. Howard had a big impact upon that realization, that sense of being prayed for by so many. Today, if someone I know has a problem and in sharing it with me I respond with, "I'll pray for you," I do it. Right then. Immediately. The power of prayer is genuine. You might never know how important it is until you become the recipient. Gail and I both felt as if we were being lifted above our trials. In fact, Gail described it as a sense of *floating*.

Howard provides access to Him via His Son and invites us to come boldly to Him. Hebrews 4:16 tells us, "Let us therefore come boldly unto the throne of grace, that we may obtain mercy, and find grace to help in time of need." And again, in Philippians 4:6, "Be careful for nothing; but in everything by prayer and supplication with thanksgiving let your requests be made known unto God." Gail and I not only prayed but were overwhelmingly supported by faithful friends who did so on our behalf. Howard moved in response to those petitions, and He literally carried us.

As proof of the power of prayer, I offer this evidence. While in Houston after confirmed diagnosis of Second Cousin Stanley—the visit that resulted in amputation of my right leg— Gail and I spent a lot of time in a local hotel after surgery. We'd frequently see the same hotel staff and guests every day. One particular day, Gail went to the hotel laundry to do a little catchup on our wardrobe cleaning, and I trailed behind in my wheelchair. An elderly black man was also in the tiny laundry room.

We exchanged greetings, and after a while, the gentleman turned to us and said, "You know, I've been watching you two."

We smiled and replied, "You have?"

He reaffirmed that he'd been watching us for days. He further explained that he was a retired physician and was at M.D. Anderson for his wife's cancer treatments.

He then said, "What is it?" We didn't know immediately what he was referring to and questioned what he meant. "What is it about you two—you have almost, well, like an aura about you." Gail and I smiled a bit awkwardly. The gentleman continued, "Clearly, you've gone through something significant here, but yet you have such obvious joy. What is it?"

Gail and I both, almost in unison, replied, "It's the Lord and all the people praying for us."

He smiled and replied, "I thought so! That's the only way, isn't it?"

Well, as far as I know, neither Gail or I have personal auras that we project—either individually or as a couple. The only explanation is the power of Howard's love—His peace that surpasses all understanding, unleashed by the faithful prayers of so many back home.

Another rather ironic Howard-directed episode involves my son Mike and his family. As I related previously, many years prior, I had turned down a rep assignment to Houston with Caterpillar. After my retirement, my son Mike moved home to Illinois and, of all things, joined Caterpillar. He had worked for them for several years when the company asked him to move his family for a rep's position. Where? The Houston office, of course! Unlike me, Mike willingly took the opportunity, and during our numerous trips to M.D. Anderson, we were able to routinely visit Mike and Sarah and three grandkids. Without Howard's intervention, we'd have missed them immensely. With Howard's direction, we all enjoyed our Houston experience together! Amazing grace!

With just those few minor *Howard Moments* as evidence of His presence (there are far too many to detail), I'd like to share how Howard also moved mightily as a result of Stanley in two wonderful ways with my sister and with my brother. I will circle back to my sister, Cindy, for the first example.

You'll recall her rather destitute state when I first met her after so many years of estrangement. After our initial reunion, she no doubt became panicked about their troubling financial state, thinking money would be their salvation. She called, begging me for a check for $20,000.

"This could help us out a lot," she pleaded. "We can make a big dent in our debt, and Jerry's looking hard for work."

I deferred at that initial call, telling her I'd pray about it. I know that response frustrated her.

Realizing her desperate need, I spoke to my brother about her plight. At the time, due to her dependence on drugs and alcohol, my brother felt that supplying direct financial support in the form of cash might only lead her and her husband, Jerry, to further pursue their habits.

"In a battle," he said, "the first casualty is truth. And in her state, I don't trust her to be responsible with cash." I had to partially agree. Cash support directly into their hands seemed risky.

So, I prayed about it a lot and concluded that if I could provide financial support each year to a few charities that I know very little about, I could certainly and *should* certainly support my sister. So, without any detail of the support given because I'm not looking for accolades here, I'll just say Gail and I helped Cindy and Jerry get back on their feet and out of debt. We purposely did not give them cash but rather worked directly with car loan companies, cell phone providers, various creditors, landlords, and the like. More important than the financial support, we strongly encouraged Cindy (and she agreed) to seek out a local church as a support network. She did so, and things actually began looking up.

A few years later, however, there was a setback. Cindy broke her pinky finger in a fall. She went to the emergency room and, regrettably, had to have surgery to set and pin the bone. It was a very nasty break. During her stay in the hospital, she developed a severe staphylococcus infection, which led to sepsis. That was brought under control, thankfully, but even after discharge, she was on intravenous antibiotics. She was on them for over six months— delivered through a medical port surgically implanted in her chest. I kept in touch with her during that timeframe, and I could sense the onset of her depression. I could hardly blame her, but I didn't realize how debilitating that depression had become. After six months, the port was removed, and the course of antibiotics was complete. Cindy had the wisdom to admit herself to a psychiatric ward to deal with her depression, afraid that she would again seek refuge in the placebos of alcohol and drugs.

In the hospital once again, she developed severe stomach cramps and suffered with them for several days. A few on-call doctors checked her over, reporting that it was most likely a passing thing. She was in the psych ward for about a week and was discharged to return home. Over that weekend (and I did speak with her), she continued to complain of severe stomach cramps, diarrhea, and significant nausea. At times, she told me she would double over in pain.

After a full weekend of suffering, she again returned to the hospital on Monday, January 18th. They admitted her immediately and ran a series of tests. The verdict? She had contracted another infection in the psych ward known as C-diff (*Clostridioides difficile*). Her immune system had been so compromised, her body simply could not muster an adequate defense.

C-diff is bad news. It's a bacterial disease that causes severe diarrhea and inflammation of the colon. Cindy's birthday is January

22nd, and I told her that Gail and I would be coming down to see them that week, as I had a consulting gig in Ft. Worth.

I also told her, "Hurry up and get well; try to get discharged by your birthday, and we'll host you for a wonderful birthday dinner on Saturday."

She said she'd do her best and she was looking forward to it.

We were traveling to Texas by automobile. On Wednesday, I received a call from Cindy's husband, Jerry, reporting that things were taking a turn for the worse.

"How bad is it?" I asked Jerry, thinking that only our dinner plans would be altered.

Jerry said, "I'm not sure Cindy's going to make it."

What a jolt that was! How could this be happening? I had only recently heard good news from Cindy, that she and Jerry had recommitted their lives to Christ and were attending church again. They were back on top of their financial situation. Jerry had found employment and due to being clean from drugs and alcohol was enjoying his new job and doing well. But now this? I couldn't process it. I just kept the car pointed toward Texas and prayed that Cindy would recover.

On the day I arrived in Fort Worth, the day before Cindy's 52nd birthday, I received another call from Jerry. Cindy had passed. On the weekend we were to celebrate her birthday, we buried her.

As sad as that was—as painful as the flood of memories and regrets were as we laid my sister to rest—Howard was there for me. He comforted me. Cindy had recommitted her life to Christ. I take no credit for anything in that transformation. It was all Howard, but I can't help but think of four years prior when Howard sent me to Houston and compelled me to reconcile with my sister. I can't help but marvel at His directing my path and Cindy's to get right with one another and to get right with God. She had many issues and was coming to grips with them. Howard took her home, a far better ending than dying in misery in a drug-laced, alcohol-induced fog.

I don't know why Howard chose to take Cindy home rather than permit her to recover fully and remain with her family. I am supremely comforted that Howard holds her safely in heaven now—absent that lingering pain, absent the depression that so often plagued her, and free from the need for artificial coping methods of alcohol and drugs. To deny Howard's impact in this situation is irrational. I see His presence. It is clearly evident. I see His grace. I see His mercy. I see His divine intervention in orchestrating the outcome. I am greatly humbled by it. All glory to God, and, "Yay, Howard!"

But Howard wasn't through with my family. For the second example of Howard's mighty work, I'll need to reintroduce you to David, my brother. Dave was the intellectual of our family. He was the smart one. Graduating very high in his class from Western Illinois University, he was an Air Force veteran, a CPA, and, ultimately, chief financial officer of a multi-national company based in South Carolina. David was also my best friend.

Whatever dysfunction plagued our family and our parents' marriage, it did not corrode the close bond that David and I shared. We liked almost all the same things, right down to our favorite candy bar—*Pay Day*—and our favorite home-cooked dinner of chicken and slickers (large homemade noodles). David and I, despite the distance between us, did a lot together. We rode motorcycles together, fished, hiked, hunted fossils, carved wood, and made Native American art. The only thing we didn't share together was a faith in Jesus Christ.

My cancer, Stanley, hit David hard. We were very, very close, and I know he feared the Big C because of our family's history with the disease. I know he also feared losing his best friend, and I did my best to reassure him. But David didn't have a faith to comfort him. He only saw the downside, not the hope that comes from faith in Howard.

I had spent well over forty years of my life arguing with David about faith. He, being the intellectual, could always find some argument that I, his intellectual second, couldn't overcome. As I mentioned previously, he even almost persuaded me in some of our far-out musings.

David was always searching, as he said, for the "smoking gun of Christianity"—ultimately proving it as myth. I made a big mistake trying to engage David on an intellectual basis. Of course, you know that was my motif, though. I tried to muscle everything in life, so it's natural that I would try to muscle through our debates. But I was never successful. I never won a single debate. Some were draws, perhaps, but many David won, and I felt helpless to nudge him in the direction of a saving faith.

You may remember that I mentioned my boys and I were at one point attempting to tackle movie production. I had written a screenplay in my Bradley University master's program. Rob Prescott had encouraged me to take a screenwriting class because the writing approach is so vastly different in style and technique. The assignment for the semester was to write at least twenty pages of a representative screenplay. I wrote 143 pages—a complete screenplay. I actually wrote it from an idea I'd tossed around in my mind for many years. More importantly, I wrote it for my brother. I was, once again, attempting to tackle the debate we continually had on the topic of faith.

I don't need to provide a full synopsis of the film here but will simply say that we considered it a Christian faith-based film. Yet it was gritty. It was a gritty detective genre film called *Out of the Heart*. The title is derived from Matthew 15:19, "For out of the heart proceed evil thoughts, murders, adulteries, fornications, thefts, false witness, blasphemies." In other words, out of man's unconverted heart is nothing but sinful will.

The logline of the film was as follows: *"Following the apparent heart attack and death of a controversial radio talk-show host, a cynical detective's nagging hunch that sinister forces are at play, drives him to doggedly pursue a killer only he is convinced exists."* Through the course of the film, this detective becomes friends with a Christian, and their encounter changes him profoundly. By the end of the story, that cynical detective finds something far more precious to believe in and, more importantly, acts upon it.

For me, this was clearly targeted at David. It wasn't a gooey-soft Christian feel-good flick. The characters were flawed, imperfect, and sinful. I knew a goody-goody film would simply chase David away. It would only confirm his contention that all Christian films sucked—filled with unrelatable characters and Christian feel-good pablum. Our film was a stark contrast to that formula. It was a serial killer who-done-it, which both he and I loved to watch, but it was ripe with Christian influence. One scene even featured a debate between a priest and a cynical talk show host on the subject of faith. The dialogue from that scene came almost verbatim from a late-night text exchange David and I had had on the same subject. "What's the opposite of faith?" I'd asked him.

"Doubt," he'd replied.

"No," I said, "faith and doubt are the same thing."

We tossed this around in debate fashion for quite a while—with David finally agreeing with my contention that faith and doubt are both *beliefs.* Only certainty is the opposite of both. And absent certainty, we all operate on some basis of belief. In fact, I told David it took more faith to be an atheist than it took to believe in God and Jesus Christ.

I prayed he'd see himself in the film and especially in that scene. He did. And the impact, he said, was profound. It caused him to think—my goal. It also caused him to seriously consider again the case for faith. At the same time, Howard was impressing upon me that this whole years-long debate was **not** a matter for the intellect but rather a matter of the heart. Duh! Considering the movie was called *Out of the Heart,* you'd think I would have gotten that message years before. It took me a long, long time to realize that—and to realize I needed to get out of Howard's way. So, ultimately, I did. I got out of Howard's way. And He did the rest.

One day, during one of David's many month-long visits, he accompanied me to have my vehicle serviced, and he noticed pocket-sized New Testament and Psalms Bibles free for the taking in the dealership's customer lounge. He took one. I said nothing. That night, he began reading. I know he did because the next morning he told me so. I said something lame like, "Good for you, bro."

Over and over I would see him reading, and he would ask me questions. If it was something I knew, I would give an answer. If it was something over my intellectual head, I would simply say, "David, I don't know, but while I don't have an answer, it doesn't impact my faith. I simply believe."

I took David to breakfast one day with a dear friend and past minister from my church. His name was Dr. Bob Pflederer. Bob, Dave, and I discussed David's questions at length over the meal. But I noticed that Bob wasn't saying much—he was just acknowledging David's comments. Dave would ask a question, and then he would pause, met with Bob's (and thankfully my) silence. After a moment or two, David would answer his own question. It was obvious he had been in the Word. He was working through his questions. Clearly, Howard was helping him find his own answers in Scripture.

After a long period of time, my brother ceased his questioning and asked Bob, "Well, whattaya' think?"

Bob smiled and replied, "David, I think you know the answers."

David began going to church in South Carolina after that. He attended adult Sunday school every Sunday, despite the fact that his spouse and adult kids did not join him. He told me often of his weekly lessons and the questions he had asked and how he felt it challenged his group and perhaps made them uncomfortable. He feared they thought he was a rebel and a challenge to their simplistic faith. I told him Howard perhaps put him in that position for a reason and to just continue being inquisitive.

"God wants our intellect to engage with Him," I said. "But he wants our heart to believe."

Unfortunately, in April of 2017, just over a year beyond Cindy's unexpected passing, David, too, developed a health problem. Gail and I were with him, hiking in Congaree National Forest in South Carolina, a place we frequently hiked. Dave began complaining that his right leg was dragging a bit. He was having real trouble navigating the trail. We terminated the hike and returned as gingerly as we could to his car. I urged him to see a doctor. He did so, and the news was not good. He had Stage IV lung and spinal cord cancer.

I returned home, and although we talked frequently, it was several weeks since I had last seen him. The cancer spread alarmingly quickly. By July of 2017, he was paralyzed from the hip down and confined to a bed.

He'd been cooped up in hospital and rehab facilities essentially since I left in April. In early July, to his supreme delight, he was discharged and went home. I decided to go visit him the weekend of July 13th, 2017. He was in a hospice bed in his home, and for the entire three days of my visit, we talked and reminisced and simply enjoyed one another's company— never leaving that room. It was his man cave, a place he loved to be, and I was thankful he was in surroundings that made him happy. But it was painful to see my brother atrophy to a mere wisp of the man he had been. Painful to know this was his last hike. Arms and legs without any muscle, it seemed. Mere skin and bones. David was wasting away to nothing, although he maintained his clever wit. We had a blessed time.

At one point, just before I left, I went to his bedside and said, "David, you know this— this body—is not you. It's only a shell of you."

He looked at me, reached out for my hand, and clasped it. He said, "I know, bro. I just can't wait to add my voice to the heavenly choir."

I kissed him on the forehead and told him I loved him.

He replied, "I love you too, bro."

It was our last conversation.

I'd lost my sister just the year prior and now was losing my brother—my best friend. A guy I'd argued with for over forty years had just claimed his dying hope—to be with Jesus in heaven, singing in the angelic choir. I was ecstatic, despite my anguish. Don't tell me Howard isn't amazing! David had accepted Christ, repented of his sins, and believed that Jesus was his Savior. Once again, *Yay, Howard and Amen!*

I flew home on the 15th of July and sent a text to Dave to let him know I'd reached home safely. I heard nothing back. Nor did I get a reply on the 16th. On the 17th, I called his son Eric, my nephew. Eric told me that Dave had slipped into a coma the day I left and was unconscious, the very day I'd left to return home. Just a week or so later, the next call came. Eric told me, amidst tears, that David had died peacefully in his sleep.

I was now the last man standing in our nuclear family. It was a sobering realization. And I thought I was already on borrowed time because of my dad's proclamation that no male relative lived past sixty. Well, David had made it to sixty-eight, and I was still kicking, even while Stanley was protesting in my right leg.

Despite those musings, of the utmost importance to me was the realization of David's peaceful abode in heaven. I marveled that Howard had demonstrated how He could use this thing called cancer—my very personal experience with Stanley—to reach not only me but to reach my very lost sister and my previously hard-hearted brother.

To the skeptic reading this, it might be suggested that my faith has willfully created an impact of Howard in all these events, that they could just as easily be explained by chance. They might believe I've derived an artificial conclusion from the circumstances and merely hoped that it was Howard directing each and every outcome. Learning from my experience with David, for the skeptic, I will simply get out of Howard's way and pray that this story is received with an open heart, instead of intellectual suspicion.

For me, Howard's presence was very real. I'm convinced. This had been Howard's story, Howard's direction, Howard's impact. And it was Howard's directed will, played out in us three siblings. As a result, knowing my sister and brother are saved and with Christ in heaven, I can only conclude that for me, Stanley was not only a gift, but he was undeniably worth it.

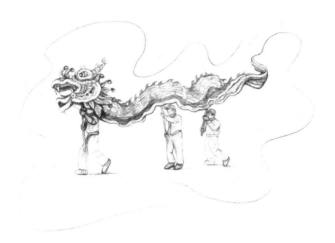

9

M.D. ANDERSON VS. STANLEY – TAKE ONE

Howard is the premier character in my story, and I fear I did not do justice to explain His impact. He was not only present in the ways previously described, He was also intimately involved in each surgery—the first of which took place February 28th, 2012.

We went to Houston a week before the surgery date. Days were filled with mind-numbing tests, pokes, and prods. Our days were free after such tests, and a couple of our kids came down to Houston to be with Gail and me. We stayed at a local hotel, and the kids stayed nearby. We did get around a bit for dinners out together or for a little sightseeing. And they stood by Gail during and after my surgery. Thankfully, I was discharged within the week.

Post-surgery, one particular episode clearly stands out in my memory. We left the hotel one evening, headed to the great salad bar at Whole Foods for something other than hotel (and thankfully) hospital chow. I was still tasting that metallic memory of hospital food and hoping for something better. I was ambulatory without a walker, albeit slow and a bit tentative. I hated that walker anyway and had always vowed I'd never use one of those tennis ball cushioned things. I only used it one day, the day following surgery, and then put it aside in favor of slowly limping and gimping along.

In the Whole Foods' parking lot, there was some sort of festive celebration going on. We noticed one of those long, snaking red Chinese dragons coursing through the lot. There were probably no less than fifteen pairs of feet beneath the dragon, powering it along on its sinuous path. Near the entrance to the store, the dragon snaked a bit too close to us, and my sweet youngest daughter, Molly, bolted to the head of the beast and screamed, "Sir, Sir! This man just had major surgery. Back off! Back off!" We all laughed and cracked up—but Molly's warning worked. The multiple feet beneath that slithering dragon did indeed back off, and we entered unimpeded. We still laugh at the scene, however, never knowing if the people inside that dragon knew English or understood a word she said. Little Molly had single-handedly defeated the *Red Devil!* It was frightened off by this mad, screaming woman! It was so very sweet of Molly to protect her father in that way, and that's how I felt throughout this first Stanley operation. I felt protected. Having a few of my kids on-hand was wonderful, and I thank Howard for the blessings of a loving family.

With regard to that first surgery, I desperately wanted to see what Stanley looked like after he was removed. Dr. Torres obliged, taking several photographs for me. Stanley was actually somewhat contained in a sort of membrane and looked like a very healthy two-and-a-half-pound roast. The doc explained that Stanley was, in fact, enclosed in a membrane, looking like five or six nodules, the size of large grape clusters—except for a small black patch near one of Stanley's edges. That, Dr. Torres explained, was the portion of the tumor killed by the chemo and radiation. Wow! It was so small! To think that twenty-five days of radiation and four weeks of chemo produced such a limited effect on Stanley clearly confirmed that he was a tough little bugger. Perhaps he was as hard-headed as the *hardened guy* I'd once projected as me.

Tough or not, chemo's ineffectiveness caused me to question its value as a weapon in my arsenal. "Shoulda' Coulda' Woulda'!" If I had it to do over again, I would definitely skip that portion of the protocol, and I expressed as much to Dr. Torres. She replied that I wouldn't likely have to endure it again. In fact, it turns out they'd decided I couldn't take radiation again due to the damage caused to good tissue. Chemo would also likely be limited for reasons of efficacy. This, to me, was no small Howard blessing!

While Stanley came out easily, there were those dubious positive margins. Stanley was very close to the femoral artery and touching the sciatic nerve. To protect leg functionality and to avoid risks to the artery, they'd elected to close me up, knowing there were still live Stanley cells present. We were informed of this, of course, and were simply told the likelihood of recurrence was almost certain at some point.

However, the biggest issue I recollect from the first surgery was the memory of my mother's passing from cancer so many years before. I remember that she went into the hospital for a simple gallbladder surgery. When they opened her up, they found inoperable esophageal cancer. They closed her back up and reported to us there was nothing more they could do. She had twelve to eighteen months to live.

When Mom came out of recovery and was wheeled to her hospital room, we three kids (Dave, Cindy, and I) were there. We rallied around her bed and encouraged her, but Mom was somewhat of a glass-half-empty person. I understood that because she had experienced a very difficult life as an orphan and foster child. She could not accept nor embrace our words of encouragement. Instead, she kept muttering she was going to die. She would drift in and out of consciousness, muttering the same words, over and over again. We could feel the fear and anxiety in her voice. At times, her tears would spill.

She said, almost as if a last wish, "You kids stay close and love one another and love Jesus." Other than that, she did not exhibit the least little bit of optimism in either word or expression. She was obviously giving up. I remember her pained appeal to love one another and to love Jesus. She had sufficient will to express her love and concern for us.

Troubled by her mental state, I spoke to the doctor and asked him about it. I also asked him if it was true that when you open up a person and find cancer, it then tends to grow more aggressively and become increasingly lethal. I'll never forget what he said: "The only thing I opened up cancer to was to your mother's mind and her will. She has to want to live."

Mom was discharged days later and went to my sister's home, essentially in a hospice situation. She was expected to fully recover from her surgery and could expect to live a good life for at least a year, maybe more.

Mom died eleven days later. The last words I heard her say were for us to *stay close and love one another and love Jesus.* Sadly, for a long period of time, I did not fulfill her dying request. Howard's plan restored that pledge with frequent trips to Texas and my reunion with sister Cindy and the ultimate salvation of my brother, David. My mom's dying wish came to my mind. I guess in His way, Howard made that wish a reality. Clearly, He was using Stanley.

Following Stanley resection number one, I recalled that episode at Mom's hospital bedside. I was determined that my will would remain strong and positive. Of course, I knew that Howard's will might be different, but as I said, I would win either way—live or die—so I was at peace. Truthfully, I felt pretty good following surgery. I shed the narcotics quickly, after only four days. I had a cumbersome drain installed and a nasty long incision some ten inches in length on the back of my thigh. But it was dressed protectively, and I could walk—albeit slowly and with a considerable limp.

Wound care became a considerable nuisance. Gail had to become my home nurse, and to her credit, she did an awesome job changing dressings every day. It was pretty gross. She'd need to empty my drain bag twice a day, dealing with all that nasty, bloody serous fluid. Apparently, I'm a big producer. There was a big cavity in the back of my leg where Stanley had once resided, and fluid trying to fill that void is very normal. That was why a drain was inserted.

Gail was constantly worried about introducing infection or otherwise harming me or delaying healing, but she was a genuine trooper. Beyond the hassle of drain management, Gail had to look at a very gross wound. She could see the muscles in my leg, pulsing and exposed all along the length of that roughly ten-inch open wound. I would turn with my back to a long closet mirror and look at Stanley's wound myself. Even to me it was gross. But Gail cared for it faithfully, and it finally showed signs of healing.

After eight months or so, while most of Stanley's former abode had healed, there remained a hole about the size of a little finger in the very tip of the closing wound. I could stick a special six-inch-long Q-tip into that cavity, and it would nearly completely disappear. I learned this is called a *sinus*. It is essentially an open track that extends from the surface of the wound to the underlying wound cavity. Being nearly six inches in depth, it was clear that Stanley's wound had not healed properly. This sinus was still producing serous drainage. We were unsure whether we should continue treatment on our own or seek medical advice.

At Gail's encouragement, I finally did contact the M.D. Anderson medical team. They referred me to the local wound clinic in Peoria. There a doctor examined the wound, concluding that the best course of action would be to slice the wound back open from the point of that open sinus. Like a spring that been under tension, the side walls of the scar tissue from the wound split apart about four inches wide. Gail continued to treat the newly reopened and just as gross wound. I visited the wound clinic once a week for various lymphatic treatments using thigh to foot wraps, as well as a fancy lymphatic drainage and massage machine. Finally, after fourteen months, the wound from Stanley's first removal closed.

During the time at home, life went on pretty much as normal. Unless I told you, you'd never know I had cancer. We went back to Houston every three months for about a year. Then every four months in year two. In year three, four, and five, we were only required to visit every six months. At the nearly five-year point, I had that initial statistic in mind that Dr. Liu had mentioned, that the survival rate for soft-tissue sarcoma was fifty percent at five years. I thanked Howard for being on the winning end of those statistics.

Then in August 2017, almost exactly five years following the initial diagnosis , we visited M.D. Anderson for one of our routine follow-ups. Unfortunately, we got some news we were hoping to avoid.

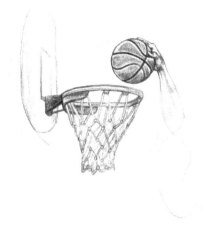

10

M.D. ANDERSON VS.
STANLEY – TAKE TWO

S tanley had returned, but round two versus Stanley was much easier. It seemed like a non-event...a slam dunk, so to speak. I remember earlier in my appointments with Dr. Torres, she discussed one of her current patients with the same type of cancer as Stanley. Trying to both calm me but also inform me that the prospects of recurrence were very real, she mentioned that this particular patient had already undergone nine surgeries. It was 2017, five years since the initial diagnosis of Stanley.

I turned to Dr. Torres and said calmly, "Okay, so this is Stanley number two—his first cousin—and he's recurred five years post-Stanley number one. Nine surgeries at five years apart each would be, let's see, forty-five years. I'll be 110 years old! Okay, I like those odds."

She smiled briefly but got back to business discussing next steps. She told us she intended to be very aggressive with Stanley's removal. She wanted to achieve negative margins and would do whatever she could to achieve them. We asked about the sciatic nerve and artery, and she told us she'd have a surgical team assembled with specialties in vascular and neurosurgery prepared to address any issues. We were confident.

Candidly, I viewed Cousin Stanley (as the grandkids called him) as a mere bump in the road. I thought it would be one final step on the journey to full recovery, cancer-free. I can't fully explain my confidence, except again for Howard's peace that surpasses all understanding and also, as in the past, the many, many prayers offered on our behalf. In truth, I just felt supremely confident about this particular surgery.

It actually went fine, this time removing an adult-sized fist of Stanley tissue. Doc Torres had indeed been aggressive, and I had a very large wound on the rear of my thigh. It was shorter in length, but broader in width. Gail and I were old pros at wound management by this time, and at least I was confident it would heal more quickly than big Stanley. The surgeon cautioned me about my optimism, however, as severely radiated tissue heals a bit slower.

And by the way, there were positive margins yet again.

I really can't complain much about any aspect of Cousin Stanley's removal in operation number two. As I said, it was pretty much a slam dunk, non-event. Except perhaps for the skin graft. Two large-size bacon strips of skin were removed from the same right leg and used to cover the wound left by Cousin Stanley's departure. Unfortunately, a nurse made a slight error allowing me to shower (at my urging), and in doing so, I got the protective film covering the graft wet. A day or so following my very sublime shower, it was clear the graft would not take. They removed the now-dead skin and bandaged me normally.

Those two strips of bacon wounds were far worse than the tumor wound. It was like severe road rash, and once it scabbed over, every time I moved, it felt like a scab busted loose and pulled and tugged at the wound that was trying to become skin. It caused both severe pain and bleeding. In a word, skin grafts are miserable. Still, with Gail's good wound care management, the bacon strips healed, and Cousin Stanley's wound closed fully after just six months.

Life at home following Cousin Stanley's removal was pretty normal, too. Except that Gail had become somewhat of a health food Nazi—determined that I would eat my way to cancer-free health. I honestly believe with all the podcast seminars she's listened to, she likely has the equivalent of a master's degree in nutrition. Eating healthy became her singular focus, and she was as determined as determined could be to get me healthy and cancer-free. It actually caused her a lot of stress because, well, I liked my junk food. I would go on my errands around lunch time just to stop off at some fast food joint and eat my junk. She knew it somehow, and it drove her crazy!

She preferred I drink these purple or brownish-green morning shakes with the consistency of mud. The ones made with good sounding fruits but always with kale or spinach or some other mystery ingredient that invariably turned the concoction an ugly brownish-green and tasted nothing like banana. These *drinks*, as she called them, poured into a glass like slowly-setting concrete.

"Here," she'd say, thrusting some dreadful-looking thick liquid toward me. "Spinach, kale, cucumber, and seeds. Drink it!"

Total yuck, but to keep peace, I complied, struggling many times to get it down. Later in my day, around lunch time, it *was all about finding Taco Bell!*

Now Gail always made great soups, and I actually do call her the *Soup Queen.* Eating healthy soup dinners was no problem; I loved them. Salads are okay, too, if they don't have every conceivable crunchy vegetable from the fridge in them. I prefer simple salads—the kinds with a bit of lettuce, lots of cheese and bacon, and scoops of blue cheese dressing. What I got was crunchy cauliflower, broccoli, celery, radishes, and carrots—***nothing*** that should be allowed to adorn a leafy lettuce salad.

Gail's degree in nutrition was admirable but in turn for me, was somewhat of a hassle. I don't know if diet alone would have ever killed Stanley, but despite my protests, it didn't kill me either. Most importantly, it pacified my wife. You know, Howard's just gotta' love her.

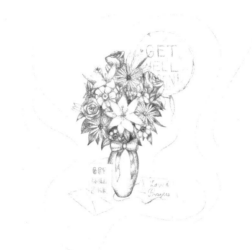

M.D. ANDERSON VS. STANLEY – THIRD TIME'S THE CHARM

O nly about fifteen months after Cousin Stanley left the building, I began to notice tingling in my right leg and especially my right foot. I developed a bit of a hitch in my *git-along* as well. Not quite a loss of balance but a tentative giving way on certain steps that didn't feel quite stable. I didn't want to admit it, but I suspected another ambush by yet another distant cousin of Stanley's. This would be, if true, Second Cousin Stanley. I really didn't want to believe his relative had taken up residence in my thigh again, but the sense of that was very real.

I fought off the urge to get checked, though. Partially because it had been a such a short time since First Cousin Stanley's extraction, and partially because I believed all versions of Stanley were relatively slow growers. Another very real reason for my reticence was that I was thoroughly fatigued of all things Houston. In fact, I'd put off two Houston check-ups in the past year because I was feeling generally terrific (minus the limp) and, again, I was Houston travel-depleted. The Houston medical team—specifically Doctor Torres—ultimately suggested, somewhat emphatically, that it was time for a follow-up visit and another MRI.

I said, "Fine," but insisted that, "an MRI in Morton is as good as an MRI in Houston. How about referring me to OSF Healthcare for a locally administered test?"

It took some jockeying back and forth, with me being on the protesting side, but in the end, M.D. Anderson yielded and issued orders for an MRI to be performed at OSF Healthcare in Morton, Illinois. Couldn't get much more local than that, and I was ecstatic. I didn't expect anything to show; I just was hoping the limp was psychosomatic and the tingling in the leg and foot were, well, my new normal caused by scar tissue pressing on the nerve. (You see, I'd read about that on the ever-faithful Internet, too. And you know, of course, if it's on the Internet, it's gotta' be true.)

In February of 2019, I had the MRI performed in Morton. I had to have disk images prepared to FedEx for my team in Houston. I sent them out late in the month, just prior to our long-scheduled trip to the Holy Land in early March. We went on that trip with about forty other wonderful people. The trip was marvelous. Eleven days' worth of great sightseeing, great food, and great fellowship. It was inspirational to be in the places where our Savior walked. But we weren't only where He walked; we walked miles and miles ourselves. I was definitely feeling it. We returned home in mid-March and after just a week's rest, took another tour in Washington, D.C., with a Christian group hosted by the Family Research Council. It was also excellent but again, a lot of walking. By this time, I knew there was an issue. It wasn't just my mind playing tricks on me; it was very likely Second Cousin Stanley.

It took M.D. Anderson a couple of months to get back to me following submission of the MRI disks. Eventually, late April, I received an email from Dr. Torres' nurse. You know it's not good news when the nurse's email opens with, "Bill, I'm so sorry to be the one to tell you this, but..." She went on to explain that the latest February MRI showed evidence that Stanley had returned, and he appeared to be "encasing the sciatic nerve." Naturally, they advised me to return right away for further testing, including their own MRI and evaluation.

Well, that was a bummer. I had no real concept of what *encasing the sciatic nerve* meant as far as functional impact longer term. I could certainly walk now. So quite naturally, I yet again turned to my expert medical advisor—the Internet. I didn't like what I found. It said such tumors were likely best treated by amputation or, more modernly, by limb-sparing surgery that would resect (cut out) the affected section of the sciatic nerve.

I did a lot of additional Internet research on quality of life after amputation and quality of life with limb-sparing sciatic nerve resection. There wasn't a tremendous amount of detail, but there was enough. I even watched a video of some other guy getting an above-the-knee amputation on YouTube. *Amazing*! Not only because a YouTube video exists on such a topic but also the surgery itself. It's astounding that surgeons can tell what they're doing with so much bloody hamburger in front of them. After all the research, I concluded one inescapable fact—this was going to be a long road.

We met with our kids and discussed this new Second Cousin Stanley and the treatment options. Most of the kids sided with Gail—have the leg amputated which would then, at least, get rid of Stanley once and for all.

"Easy for you to say," I replied, but, of course, I fully understood their sentiment.

Our trip to Houston was set for early May. We met with Dr. Torres, and she fully explained the limb-sparing surgery. Clearly, that was her preference. It would involve removing considerable muscle and tissue along with severing the sciatic nerve, removing about ten to twelve inches of it along with Stanley. I asked about leg functionality post-surgery, and Dr. Torres explained I could be mobile again in time with a brace. However, I would have no knee, leg, or foot sensation or control below the thigh. Hmmm...didn't sound too appealing.

I explained to Dr. Torres that following my right shoulder replacement in December of 2018, the worst part was the twenty-four nerve block they'd administered and the resultant dead piece of meat that was my arm. It caused so much anxiety in me that I had had a panic attack at home, fearful that I'd never regain use of my right arm again. It was extremely frightening to look at a piece of your body over which you have zero control. I freaked. I really did. Gail comforted me, expressing that I was likely severely overreacting.

But I'd had a very restless night with that dead arm, sleeping very little and continually touching the meat that was once my arm to discern if any feeling was returning. Finally, of course, that nerve block did fade by the following afternoon. Normal function and sensation returned, thank Howard! But that experience made a huge impression upon me emotionally. I hated it. Such a helpless and unnatural feeling. I couldn't *imagine* having a dead limb for life. The thought of it was more than a little frightening. It was no coincidence that Howard directed the timing of that experience. It made a great impact on my ultimate decision.

Further on in our discussions, Gail asked about amputation, and Dr. Torres said, "I certainly won't do it. If you go that route, it will have to be another surgeon, not me."

I didn't know at the time if this was just her complete refusal to consider amputation as an appropriate option or if she was just expressing that she was not the right specialist to perform such a surgery. Bottom line, we left Houston on that note, and for the next few weeks, mulled over our not-too-exciting alternatives.

To her credit, Dr. Torres also must have mulled over my expressed anxiety as well. About two weeks later, she actually called me at home in Illinois. Her call to my home was not typical, but I believe it speaks volumes about the compassion and care of the staff at M.D. Anderson. She told me that she indeed had been pondering my anxiety about the numb and *dead* limb, suggesting that I return for second opinions from two other surgeons—surgeons who had not heard of my case when presented before M.D. Anderson's Tumor Board. (Notably, surgeons present all such cases to this board—a team of excellent doctors—to ensure that their collective best thinking goes into the treatment protocol and surgical approach before any such operation. Impressive!) I told the doc that I had somewhat gotten my head around her suggested approach, but she rather strongly suggested I return to Houston just the same. I'm glad she did.

That visit occurred during the first week of June, at which time I met with a specialist in reconstructive surgery, Dr. Alex Mericli, and an orthopedic oncologist, Dr. Valerae Lewis. The purpose of both appointments was to help me understand what might lie ahead. Both docs did a deep dive into the procedures and recovery aspects of their respective approaches.

Dr. Mericli explained the approach that would be taken in the limb salvage option. Essentially, the huge cavity created by

Dr. Torres removing the muscle, surrounding tissues, a portion of my sciatic nerve, and Second Cousin Stanley, would be filled with tissue from my back. He would remove a section of my latissimus dorsi muscle—the muscle that extends, adducts, and medially rotates the humerus—the long bone in the upper arm. He would take sufficient muscle and tissue that the tissue flap would have its own blood supply, negating the need for skin grafts. (Whew! That was the only positive news thus far from this discussion.) The doctor seemed confident, and we left with a clear understanding of the limb-sparing surgery, and what we'd be up against for recovery post this iteration of Stanley's removal.

We then met with Dr. Lewis and her team. I discovered that Dr. Lewis was the head of orthopedic oncology at the University of Texas and was quite literally world-renowned. Can you see Howard at work? I certainly can. I was supposed to have an appointment with someone else, and actually, that appointment was two days after my appointment with Dr. Mericli. It would have extended my stay another two full days. At the last minute, that appointment was cancelled for reasons that were never explained. I was switched to a same-day appointment with Dr. Lewis. Okay, tell me that's not Howard!

Dr. Lewis came into the exam room with a flourish and no less than six student physicians, another physician—Dr. Alysia Kemp—and Physician's Assistant Nadia Leach. The students were trailing after her like so many goslings after a mother goose. They all squeezed into the tiny room, nearly surrounding Gail and me. Dr. Lewis was an impressive lady—confident, all business, but with an undeniable spark of great humor and wit. After brief pleasantries—the majority of which were introductions to the cast of characters assembled in the exam room—she quickly got down to business. She explained what would be involved in approaching Second Cousin Stanley with the amputation option. She looked at my scars from both previous Stanleys and suggested a total hip-disarticulation amputation would be necessary, likely due to the fact that the prior disease was fairly high in the upper thigh. In other words, amputation of the entire leg at the hip.

Sounded pretty drastic, so I pressed her. "What happens if I do nothing?" I thought that was a reasonable question since I was fully ambulatory (save for some mild numbness and tingling) when I walked to the appointment. I learned to love this quality about Dr. Lewis, her directness, that is.

She simply smiled and said, "Then you'll die from the disease."

How tragically ironic that Caterpillar wanted to send me to Houston to be *mobile* in a marketing role. Now, forty years later, Stanley brought me to Houston where I would become *immobile. Coincidence?*

She went on to explain a bit more about this version of Cousin Stanley. Clearly, this Stanley had a bit of an attitude. Instead of being enclosed in a sort of membrane, as tumors one and two were, this version of Stanley had tentacles—long, slithery fingers extending both north and south in my limb. She showed us the image on the computer screen of the most recent MRI—one done on this visit and only three months after the February MRI from Morton. Stanley was distinctly different from his prior cousins and notably larger than his prior snapshot from February. It seemed to me that if we waited on this version of Stanley, the chances of metastasis increased. We talked further about amputation and rehabilitation and what to expect. At that point, Dr. Lewis—a real no-nonsense doc—pulled out her cell phone, quickly dialing a number she knew by heart.

"Hello, Dave? Valerae here. Do you have some time this after-noon? Great! I'd like to send over a patient considering a total hip disarticulation. Great, I'll send him over." And just like that, Dr. Lewis had paved the way for me to meet the premier hip-disartic-ulation prosthetic specialist in Houston. Before we left, she said to both of us, "You two have a difficult decision to make. Think it over for a few days and let us know. We'll be here." With that, she and most of her entourage exited the room.

Except for Nadia. She, I quickly learned, was going to become my "go to" person. She's the glue that seems to hold it all together in terms of patient interaction with the surgical team. She was terrific—incredibly responsive whether by email or phone—during working hours or after hours. She was a true blessing, handling requests for everything from pain meds to driver evaluation orders to physical therapy orders. All of this was to be done remotely back in Illinois, so it was no small task for her to coordinate such things. She was amazing, and I'm so thankful she was on the team to tackle Second Cousin Stanley.

After our parting discussions with Nadia, Gail and I collected our things and left for a walk to the prosthetics specialist, just a few short blocks away. Yes, we walked. We met Mr. David Baty of Care Prosthetics and Orthotics. Dave was a very pleasant man and made us feel right at home. He did not rush. He spent over an hour with us and explained the process for constructing a prosthetic for my particular situation. He explained how he would work with me in fit up, adjustment, and training in how to effectively and safely become mobile again. He was very encouraging. It felt good. Maybe it even felt right. But it was still a big decision, and I wasn't quite there yet.

Two things Dave said really stuck with me. One was this: "You're lucky you got Dr. Lewis. She's the absolute best. Someone's looking out for you." (Can everyone say *Howard*?) The second statement that really hit me was this: "You know, Bill, when it's all said and done, you'll fight more within your head than you'll fight with a prosthetic."

That made perfect sense to me and appealed to that mental toughness side of me that still existed in my spirit and was looking for another mountain to conquer. *Mind over matter* was my frequent mantra in other tough situations. Stanley was just one more tough situation, and it sounded like a new hill to climb—not one to retreat from. This appealed to my *die trying to reach the top* mindset.

When we finished our discussions, Gail and I prepared to leave. As we exited the building, we saw it was raining rather heavily. We stepped inside and moved to the receptionist's desk to request a taxi. Dave walked out at just about that moment and said, "Oh man, it's raining. Let me drive you home." Again, talk about feeling like we were with the right folks; this was pretty amazing. Dave drove us to our hotel; we thanked him, and upon exiting Dave's truck, Gail and I said to one another, "Now that was a *Howard Moment!*"

When these two deep dive appointments were concluded, Gail and I were free to fly home. We did so, along the way unpacking and digesting all that we'd heard. I was all over the map as Gail and I discussed which path felt right. We didn't reach a conclusion in those few short hours from Houston to Peoria. At least I did not. In fact, it took me several days of processing our options.

On one hand, I'd have a leg. I wouldn't look like a freak (with apologies to all amputees—those were just my fears speaking). But it would be dead meat hanging uselessly below my thigh. I'd also still have a spot for Stanley to yet again reappear. At this point, the prospect of those nine surgeries Dr. Torres told me about didn't seem so funny.

On the other hand, if I opted for the amputation (my family's preferred option), I would have no leg at all. What would limbless life be like? I was pretty alarmed at that prospect, primarily because I'd been so independent in my life up to that point. I also had many hobbies I worked on in my basement shop, and I worried, *Would I ever be able to resume those interests? Could I handle stairs?* I was also more than a little alarmed and fearful about the prospects of never driving again. *Would driving—would getting into my vehicle safely—even be possible?*

I went back and forth. I was all for limb-sparing surgery one day and amputation the next.

A dear friend, whose husband was also undergoing cancer treatments in Houston, came up to me in church and said, "I'm jealous."

I asked why, thinking, *Why would anyone be jealous of my prospects with Stanley?*

She thoughtfully explained, "You're lucky. I wish my husband had something that could be cut off to remove his cancer."

Yeah, I thought, *it could be lots worse.*

I also circled back with sweet Dr. Liu in Peoria. I'll never forget her words as we discussed the situation and reviewed the new Stanley's MRI results. She turned to Gail and me and simply said, "I give my blessing for the amputation."

Ultimately, however, the biggest influence on my decision was Gail. I had already put her through a lot and arguably enough of Stanley and all that came with him. With her constant worry about recurrence, all the wound issues she'd managed, and all the stress and anxiety of fearing Stanley would metastasize to my lungs or liver, I knew amputation would give her the greatest peace. If removing the leg meant removing Stanley for good, then let's have at it.

I emailed Dr. Lewis and said, "I'm all in." I also emailed Dr. Torres and said, "We're opting for life over limb. Thanks for everything."

She wrote back, "You'll be in good hands."

At that moment, once the decision had been declared, Howard gave me an immediate peace. The debate was over; we were going back to Houston. *Stanley...you're toast!* A door sign flashed into my memory—one from the men's restroom on the ninth floor of the sarcoma clinic. I'd passed through it many times before. It was a large wooden Stanley door this time, with a blue and white placard picturing a silhouetted and wheelchaired figure. It simply said, "Push to Operate." Howard's sense of humor just tickles me! I'd been appropriately pushed. Time now to operate.

The church jungle drums still worked, and it wasn't long before another flood of cards, letters, emails, and texts arrived. Again, all committing to pray for us, with many showing great concern for the challenges of our road ahead. It seemed losing a limb was a really big deal—a sad deal. Amusingly, my sister-in-law said, "Amputations aren't the norm around here, Bill— Stanley's made you a celebrity!"

There was one more amazing Howard moment before we headed back to Houston for the big surgery. I had never heard of a man named Josh Stuber. Not once in my life. But three separate people asked me if I knew him, and it was in the context of Stanley and my upcoming surgery. One person was my dental hygienist. The other was my oldest son, Mike. The third was my new family physician, Dr. Trent Proehl. Trent is an amazing physician, and I don't hesitate to call him friend. All three were telling me what an amazing guy Josh was, and the kicker? Josh had experienced a total hip disarticulation amputation just the year before.

Dr. Proehl reached out to Josh (another of his patients) on my behalf and asked if he'd be willing to speak with me. Dr. Trent also encouraged me greatly and was very supportive of the decision he knew I had made. In no small way, Dr. Trent was instrumental in helping me face that choice with optimism and confidence.

That very night, I received a text from Josh, asking if he could stop by the next day. That was to be the last day before departure, the last possible day I could see him. Of course, we invited him over.

I somewhat nervously hung out in my den on the morning of our appointment, as I have windows with a view to the driveway. The first thing I noticed, and right on time, Josh drove up and got out of his car and walked to our front door, easily scaling three steps with a bright, shiny prosthetic leg. I certainly took special note of that level of independence—driving and stairs!

Once inside, the second thing I noticed was his beaming smile and total poise and confidence in his own skin. I thanked him for coming and invited him in, and we went to the living room. Gail and I sat there, all ears. Josh explained his farming accident, the fight for his life with all of the blood loss, his struggle with excruciating phantom pain, and the past year's journey with both physical therapy and fit-up for his new prosthetic leg. He was a wealth of information but, more importantly, a wealth of positivity and inspiration. He didn't sugarcoat it but nonetheless brought a level of confidence and positivity that was infectious. Before he left, he asked if he could pray for us. Notice Howard in any way? He prayed a beautiful prayer for our peace during the journey ahead, and we parted as new friends. It was again, in our minds, an amazing Howard moment.

The next day, we eventually made it to Houston. We arrived on June 18th after a long day of delayed flights and anxious waiting around crowded airports. We experienced multiple delays and instead of arriving at George Bush International airport at 7:00 pm as planned, we got in at almost midnight. Our reserved shuttle had long since departed, without us, of course, apparently not willing (understandably) to wait five hours for a $75 shuttle fare. I made arrangements to get a rental car at the counter and drove the all-too-familiar route to our hotel. To me it felt as if the transportation fairies were protesting this trip as much as I was and the demons were wreaking havoc with our travel plans. Indeed, it could be called a travel day from hell, and all aspects of travel were revolting with me against this journey back to Houston and the surgery that awaited. Again, the power of all those many prayers sustained Gail and me. Yes, I knew it would be a long road, but I was traveling with Howard, and, as Gail said, we were *floating* along our path.

On the 20th of June, we actually walked from our Houston hotel to M.D. Anderson. It was a lovely sunny morning, already foretelling the sweltering heat that would soon envelope the city. I noticed the trees, the grass, the beautiful landscaping. The flowers and plants reflected the meticulous care only an army of gardeners could muster. We passed a continual array of modern medical buildings far too quickly. This was to be my last walk on two legs, and I wanted to enjoy it. I recall looking down at my legs as we made that brief four-block walk. Everything looked good to me. What was I doing? Walking in fully ambulatory, yet knowing in a few hours, my world would be turned upside down.

We checked in at the hospital receptionist. They were ready for me, and the process of admission went very smoothly. Too quickly for my taste. Before I could even think about running away, I was in a hospital bed, getting prepped for surgery.

The surgery went quite well (according to the surgeons). I can't personally confirm that because I was sleeping throughout and didn't get to watch. I wish they had videoed it. Anyway, during prep, they gave me an epidural, and I teased about finding out what it was like to be pregnant. That's about all of the prep I remember. Before long, I was totally out of it.

The surgery was about five-and-a-half hours in length. Upon conclusion of the surgery, Stanley *had left the building*. He was gone for good, and in recovery, Dr. Lewis told me the margins were great. Finally! A bit extreme, but the margins were good. Of course, my right leg had to escort Stanley from the premises, but by amputating at the hip, the margins between good and bad tissue were large. Good thing! The only *good* tissue left on my right side was my butt. Thankfully, it's a good-sized one.

Also, thankfully, the medical team expressed great confidence that risk of metastasis was very low, as was the probability of any recurrence. Once again, Howard and the power of prayers were with us.

The surgeons also confirmed that Stanley had indeed grown multiple tentacles extending into cavities of my leg far more so than had prior versions of Stanley. Hearing the surgeon's report confirmed to me that Stanley was trying to get out of hand—what better way than by growing *fingers*. Bottom line—the surgeons assured Gail and me that we had made the right choice to undergo the amputation. Stanley's prior surgeon, Dr. Torres, sent flowers to our hospital room that very day. Her card said she was wishing us well and again confirmed we were in good hands.

Okay, so what was the first week like without having a leg below the hip bone? Honestly, it felt very much like still having a leg—albeit an extremely painful one. Seriously, I could still feel my total leg, from hip to toes. Thigh, knee, calf, foot, toes...it was like they were all still attached. The only issue was that the nerves that would normally supply movement and sensation to it were in hostile rebellion. Through a phenomenon known as Phantom Limb Pain (PLP), my leg was very vehemently reminding me of its connection to my brain. Of course, it wasn't really there, but I couldn't tell my brain that. Between grimaces, I marveled at that phenomenon and how amazingly and wonderfully we are constructed by the Creator.

Phantom Limb Pain was the worst pain I've ever felt. I mean **The Worst**. (With a nod to women who deliver babies, of course.) It took a few days to figure out the right dosage and frequency for the narcotics to keep ahead of the pain without making me too loopy. For the most part, they achieved that balance. When the scale tipped, I tipped it toward pain over being loopy. I can manage pain, but I can't manage loopy. And I was fearful of those recurring hallucinations.

After just a week in the hospital, they were talking **discharge**. There were some hoops to go through, and I wasn't sure I'd be released, but on the seventh day following Stanley's demise, I was discharged. I think that's pretty amazing. Again, I thanked Howard and the many offering prayers for my swift recovery.

I went back to the hotel, where Gail had been holed up for the week, and it was there that I began this narrative. It was good to be free of the hospital setting, even though our hotel room wasn't much larger. It still produced a feeling of freedom. I was feeling very much at peace with the decision and received a lot of encouragement from friends and family. I must also declare that the nursing staff at M.D. Anderson are wonderful people, too—very caring and clearly with many believing folks who likewise encouraged me.

Spending two weeks in the hotel became tedious. But we got around as much as we could, interlaced with a lot of rest and Gail having to empty my bloody drain at least twice a day. The hotel staff became very familiar to us, and we engaged with them in a fun and playful manner. No doubt, I think our demeanor was a bit puzzling to them. We spoke openly of Stanley and our journey, with lots of opportunity to speak of being sustained by Jesus. There were several *Amens* and many nodding heads. We discussed prayer, faith, and the temporal nature of life and its challenges. We also encouraged the need to focus more on the eternal. In our view, we made many friends among the hotel staff. One dear employee even gave us both going away presents—a beautiful handmade blouse for Gail and a print of the State Flag of Texas for me. It was very touching, and, again, I'm confident was directed by Howard.

While at the hotel, I had to commence my physical therapy. Read that as a major *ugh*. It was difficult and frustrating. I was pushed gently to expand my capabilities and learn to cope, even conquer, my new limitations. I had a great physical therapist, Alex Penny. He had a great sense of humor, and I liked him immediately. I would come in with the right pants leg in a knot, asking Alex if my right knee looked swollen. "It's *knot*, you know?"

He'd chuckle and say, "Yeah, now get on the bike; we'll work it out."

On another occasion, I came in with my pants leg unknotted. I said, "Hey, Alex, I've been working out." Then I'd toss my right empty pants leg over my good leg and exclaim, "See? Look how easy it is to cross my legs now!"

We had a blast together, if exercising could ever be called fun, and he encouraged me to push myself and build up my core in anticipation of the new prosthetic to come. We were on a mission, which we dubbed *Seeking the Six Pack*.

He'd tell me, "It's in there, man; we just have to find it!"

I also had a great occupational therapist, Leslie Ott. She was instrumental in helping me upgrade to a much lighter, much more mobile wheelchair—even allowing me to specify Chicago Cubs blue. She exhibited tremendous patience and empathy, and I appreciated her immensely. Those three weeks, despite the lingering sense of confinement, went pretty quickly. We were back and forth to M.D. Anderson facilities for follow-up visits, PT, and even acupuncture treatments.

Acupuncture treatments, while kind of zen-like, were amazing and very helpful in controlling the phantom pain. I felt none at all when those five needles were stuck into my right ear and into several of my left foot's toes. There were several other weird and seemingly unrelated places on the body that received punctures—twenty-one in all. I'll tell you what, immediately following acupuncture, the pain was back, raging as ever. Too bad I couldn't walk around pierced with all those needles. I still needed the drugs and had some nasty nights. Gail was my doting nurse, and we managed.

On the 12th of July, we had a final appointment before being released to return home. Dr. Kemp removed the sutures, and praise be to Howard, Dr. Lewis ordered the drain removed. Free at last! Gail and I made reservations to return home the next day. We flew non-stop from Houston to St. Louis, and my eldest daughter, Erin, with husband, Ross, picked us up at Lambert Field. We were finally returning home.

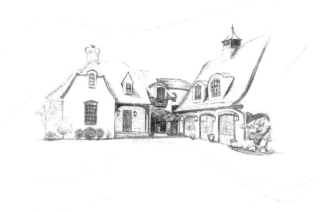

HOME AGAIN, HOME AGAIN – JIGGITY-JIG

W e arrived home from St. Louis a little bit before midnight. All in one piece—well, minus one piece. Son-in-law Ross helped me navigate the stairs from the garage into our home, freaking Gail out by my very cumbersome entrance. But I made it in the door, and, finally, we were really home. In the fridge, we found an amazing food gift basket, sent from dear former work colleagues in New York—ironically, where my journey with Stanley began. A fitting denouement. We needed a midnight snack, and the fridge was empty, save for this amazing food basket. Again, don't tell me this wasn't Howard at work!

I was eager to adjust to my new norm. Hopefully, my *temporary* new norm. There is still the hope of a prosthetic that will restore much greater mobility and the independence I hunger for. I was still very much struggling with that weird phantom pain. It was excruciating at times, as I guess my brain was still protesting what I had done to my body.

Saturday, July 13th, was my first full day home. And thus far, I had not yet had any emotional breakdown. It came, ironically at the end of my first day home. I think in my mind, the thoughts of coming home meant *normalcy*. Instead of cruising around limited space hotel rooms or hospital corridors in my walker or wheelchair, I'd be in the *wide-open spaces* of home. Where I'd feel whole again. Where pain would subside. Where I'd be navigating easily.

We had a slew of family visitors that first Saturday. All of the grandkids took turns either pushing me around in the wheelchair or taking rides in it themselves. Everyone thought it was such a cool chair, and not one seemed put off by my absent limb. Only little Caroline, aged four said, "That's weird and scary." But before long, she was sitting in my lap and giving me sweet, but short, cuddles. By nine that evening, all the family fun came to an end as everyone departed for their own homes. Gail and I were alone.

In the silence of my new digs, instead of feeling free, what I felt was the overwhelming sense that the world was indeed *larger*— yet I was even more keenly aware of my confinement and limitations. I finally broke down in tears that likely had been held in check for several weeks.

Gail consoled me, of course, but it was a difficult all-out cry. I was feeling pretty down. The phantom pain had reared its ugly head throughout the day, and I could not get on top of it. I was loath to take more narcotics because I wanted to be fully present when my family visited. When they left, all I had was my pain and my sense of limitation. I just wanted to escape my circumstances.

Gail, bless her heart, had long expected this release. I had not. She kept telling me, "It's temporary, Bill. It will get better. You're strong. We all love you. Howard has it covered."

After a while, I calmed down, somewhat ashamed because I had so much more to celebrate than to lament. We prayed, and then I wheeled myself off to bed.

In bed, I prayed again. I actually fell asleep praying earnestly—asking for forgiveness for my selfish attitude and then forgiveness for losing focus in my prayer as I was drifting off. Sometime during the night, Gail put a hand-painted canvas print by my bedside, knowing this would be the first thing I saw when I woke. That painting had been made by my granddaughter Ellie just the year prior. It was a beautiful hand-scripted rendering of one of my favorite verses, Jeremiah 29-11: "For I know the plans I have for you, declares the LORD, plans for welfare and not for evil, to give you a future and a hope."

Sunday morning, I woke up feeling better. I immediately saw and read Ellie's painting. I smiled. And my attitude was back on an even keel. I had a pretty good day. Actually, it's been good since—except (and I hate to whine) for the confounded phantom pain. It's still kicking my butt. Big time. I'm out of narcotics and really don't want to get more because of my fear of dependency. The other meds they gave me aren't even making a dent in the pain. I felt it was getting better in Houston right before we were released to come home, but it's still here, strong as ever. I guess when I wrote that I must have been high on drugs. Literally.

Just the other day, I wrote the docs in Houston because where the drain was removed, there is a developing seroma (a pocket of serum fluid under the skin). I can actually hear it sloshing around when I move. It's normal and not particularly threatening, except it does have an impact on healing time and has some risk of infection. The Houston docs said to keep an eye it, which we're doing.

I confessed to my daughter Erin that I felt as if I'd lost a significant portion of my body—you know, the temple where Howard's Holy Spirit resides. My sweet daughter simply quipped, "No, Dad. Now, you're just more concentrated." And that was the perfect metaphor for what I needed to do going forward.

I needed to *be* concentrated. Not on myself or my plight but concentrated on Howard, focused on my family and friends. Most importantly, I needed to concentrate on telling this story in a manner that gives Howard the glory.

Yes, you see, *self* still rears its ugly head in my life. But Erin said it well; I was now *concentrated*. New, full-strength Bill. Less in the physical sense, perhaps, but hopefully more keenly attuned in the spiritual sense and fully recognizing my dependence upon Howard. I had the fullness of the Holy Spirit within, just in a slightly smaller package. *Concentrated strength.*

So, that strength and grace and power and mercy of Howard and His spirit living in me—*that's* what I need to project now. That's what I need to reflect. It's not about what I accomplish. Howard's still teaching me it's not about me and it's not about achievement. I can be a stubborn learner, but I now know that it's really all about Howard. Stanley is an inconsequential bump in the road. And the road leads to eternity. It really is all about HIM. And everything I do must give the glory to Him—not seek it for myself or attempt to garner pity, sympathy, or empathy.

Bottom line, this has been a remarkable journey. Sometimes difficult but always providing a means for me to see Howard as the glorious God that He is. Full mobility will be restored. I know it. It may be a bit of a longer road than I would like, but it's a road I do not travel alone. Howard, family, and many, many dear friends have been with me on this road, and I know will continue to journey with me. Praise Howard. Praise our Great God. I could not be more grateful.

- 13 -

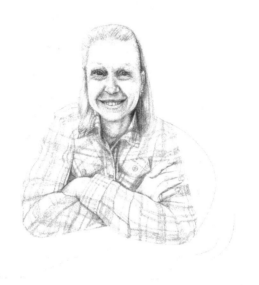

INTRODUCING GAIL

One person who intimately traveled this journey with me is my wife, Gail. I've referenced her many times in this narrative. She's been an integral part and has been by my side throughout. She obviously is an important part in the retelling of Stanley's tale, and I believe it's important to actually give voice to her unique perspective. So, I've asked her to contribute her thoughts. She's nervous about writing, but I've told her to *just be yourself*. And so, without further ado, and absent any filters or my own edits, here is the unvarnished perspective of my wife. Allow me to introduce you to Gail:

Tickets to a jazz club, the theater, and a comedy club, our favorite dinner was true Italian in Little Italy, New York City! We took the train up north of the city to a restoration furniture company, which rekindled one of our dreams, thoughts of opening a secondhand shop back home, selling nothing but our cool! We walked miles for four days and nights, loving every minute.

It was our thirty-seventh wedding anniversary and the last day of our trip. We were being lazy, lounging on our hotel bed reading the paper this beautiful sunny morning, looking forward to breakfast and catching our flight home later in the day.

"Gail, look at my leg!"

I looked in Bill's direction, my eyes landing right on the bump protruding from the inside of his right thigh. Whatever it was, it was popping out an inch, with a three-inch spread. I asked if it hurt; it didn't hurt. My blood pressure soaring, I was thinking *cancer* but said nothing. I was frantic, my mind racing; I felt helpless. *Help...help me God!* Bill acted like it wasn't a big deal; me, too. Not much was said the rest of the day, so it was a quiet plane ride home. What did this all mean? Our life was going to change, I just knew it.

We were home, and I needed a plan. Trying to choose the right words, I suggested he have that right leg looked at.

He responded, "I have a doctor appointment in a couple of months, so I'll bring it up then."

"Are you kidding me?" I freaked out after hearing that totally male comeback. "Bill, this could be serious; go now, **today**!"

After my living with panic for months, he finally went to that appointment. To make it through that wait, I finally gave it all to God, thinking, "It's Bill's body, his life." I had to give it up. I was silently angry that he thought nothing about my feelings then. I knew he was afraid, but so was I.

The doctor asked if he fell and how long had the bump been there? I remember Bill was making something and a knife had gone into that leg; it was deep. Maybe the blade hit a vessel, leaving a pool of blood from that self-inflicted knife attack.

"Let's take an MRI, give it six months, and we'll check it again with another MRI."

Well, wasn't this great? It would be a year since we found the bump. Bill loved hearing those words, "Let's give it six months."

"That's a good plan, Doc!"

In six months, that area was scanned again, and there was a change. That bump was bigger. What a tough year for me—the wait, dealing with a headstrong husband. It made me mad. It drove me insane, but I usually held it all in. Imagining what Bill might be feeling made me silent. I was sure he didn't want me telling him what to do.

So, it was a sarcoma—a cancerous tumor in the right upper thigh. Our oncologist in Peoria suggested Bill go to M.D. Anderson in Houston for treatment; they specialized in sarcomas.

"Please direct us, Lord; show us the way."

Our first visit was a frightening experience—huge hospital, many sick, sad people. Tests were taken—blood, MRI, chest X-ray, CT scan, and more. This was eight years ago, and I wonder why so many people have cancer. Before this, I never said the word *cancer*; it's a scary word, you know?

I was afraid to enter a hospital. Well, I do both now without a hitch. It seems those huge parking decks became fuller each year, more and more cancer. I asked the surgeon if Bill should follow a certain diet, and she said, "No, it has nothing to do with diet."

Ha! I knew better, as I grabbed a couple pieces of candy from the front desk. Why did a cancer clinic have candy on their counters? *Cancer loves sugar, and doctors need money, that's why!*

I do know some doctors are learning more about nutrition. It's about time. Yes, I believe good food is our best medicine.

Chemotherapy was administered in Peoria with direction from Houston. Bill had three different chemo drugs pumped into his veins constantly for a whole week while lying in the hospital. Then he spent two weeks at home. He did this schedule four times and declined the fifth, sixth, seventh, and eighth rounds because he couldn't do it one more time. He experienced terrible side effects, plus those drugs take a person to almost death, leaving the patient with a very low immune system for years. No more chemo for Bill.

Those were hard weeks, seeing Bill captive in that bed, being poisoned. The first few days we could visit and laugh together, but on day four, the drugs took him away—sleeping, feeling sick, feeling sad, feeling helpless, feeling like, *Is this all there is?*

Jesus kept my mind in check. "It's an adventure; God has this!" Through it all, prayers from family and friends were heard, and we felt peace. We are forever grateful.

There was a two-month rest before we headed south again for radiation. Twenty-eight days of radiation, one-and-a-half minutes a day at 6:30 am, excluding weekends. Let's see, what to do? Taking drives in all directions, checking out small towns, San Antonio, Austin, Galveston, malls, secondhand shops looking at furniture, frames, lamps, rugs, and chairs! Trying to keep busy for a month; this was our fun and our sanity. Our most important question each day, "Where and what's for dinner?" I felt awful that Bill was getting burned every day and I was getting good seafood every night. It was work for both of us, feeling down because of our situation but trying to be light.

"Okay, so-o-o," I asked in a happy tone, "what direction do we go today?"

Bill was going through the medical vortex, as he says, and it was a big change in his life and mine. I realize how much it has affected our children and grandchildren, family and friends. It was different for them; they had fear, questions. "Will Dad or Grandpa be okay?" It was hard for family and friends, seeing someone they love go through this.

All I can say is, I'm sorry for the fear and difference it made in your lives. I thank you all for praying for your dad, your grandpa, your family member, your friend, and for me, too! This is all happening for a reason; it always is. God knows, and adversity brings change and growth.

"Please show me, Father; help me make changes."

It was time to have Stanley removed, so down to Houston. During tests and admittance, we were wondering, "What is Stanley? How big is he?" I prayed for my Bill, in Jesus's name, that surgery would go well. I was praying for everyone and everything as I waited. Stanley was the size of a beef roast, and chemo had killed tissue the size of a dime. Chemo did nothing to his tumor but filled him with chemicals, which really bothered me. The surgeon made a ten-inch incision and told me the tumor plopped out on the table looking like five connected lemons. Bill was in the hospital a week, then the hotel for two weeks to heal before our flight home.

Home again, we settled into the healing process. He didn't want to be dependent, so he pushed. In two weeks, that incision had a one-half-inch blow out, a big setback. He was producing a lot of fluid, which settled in the open cavity where Stanley lived. The Peoria Wound Clinic enlarged the opening along his healed incision to six inches and inserted a drain. It was an open wound, the muscle sitting right there. I cleaned around the muscle, down inside his leg, then dressed it every day. It took fourteen months for the three-inch-by-six-inch incision to completely heal from the inside out. It was a long year, but Bill had a good attitude. After so many months, he was cleaning and dressing his own wound and doing a great job too.

Bill was changing, too. I could see his demeanor becoming more positive, more patient. This adversity was making him a better man—the man I always knew he could be.

In the next few years, we took many trips to Houston for checkups and were thankful for all clear tests—"No cancer!" A good dining experience always followed a happy appointment. We knew another tumor could return any time because live cancer cells were left in his leg. The bad cells were next to his main artery and the sciatic nerve—no clear margins, no complete removal.

Five years later, tumor number two had arrived. It was smaller, but the surgeon took a lot of tissue to have good margins. This wound closed up in six months, hallelujah! There were still cancer cells in Bill's leg. I lived in constant fear of recurrence, until I would remember to give it away. *God has this covered; quit wasting your time, Gail.*

Now there were twin scars, from tumor one and tumor two, on the back and side of Bill's right thigh, each ten inches or so. Also, two large dark pink stripes, skin graft scars, on the front of Bill's right thigh to cover tumor two, which didn't work because they got wet in the hospital shower. The nurse started taking the film bandage off of his leg before taking a shower.

Bill said, "No, the film should stay on while I shower!"

Water found its way under the pulled film. We didn't need that chemo, and now we didn't need to have two large pieces of skin sliced from his thigh either.

Patience, it's life, things like this happen, I thought.

The raw skin from the grafts hurt for months, worse than the big hole in his leg, but Bill was gracious, and I was amazed.

It was April 2019; Bill and I were in Israel on a wonderful tour. He could feel something was happening in his leg. It felt heavy, a little numb. Getting up into the bus was draining, and after walking for a time, he needed to sit down. Our trip was ten days long, and he was so ready to get back home.

A scheduled tour to Washington, D.C., was just a week after our return from Israel. I knew that Bill would push himself to go; it had been on the calendar for a year. My Bill is a *get done now* kind of guy—push, push! Wishing I had a little of that drive, he's my perfect partner. Again, it was wearing but a great trip. In and out of a bus, a lot of walking, and again, he was ready to get home. His right leg was swelling. We wrapped it with towels or one of his shirts, then propped it up whenever we were in the hotel. I could feel Bill was anxious and knew he wasn't sharing his true feelings. This had me worried, and I was happy to get home, too.

"We've got to see what's going on. Please, Lord, I pray it's not another tumor."

It had been less than two years, and tumor three was here and with a vengeance. Stanley had grown around the sciatic nerve and was bigger than tumor two. On the MRI, we could see the tumor was stretching out and heading north and south in his thigh. I felt panic again.

"Let's get it out, now!"

The sarcoma surgeon wanted to save the leg by cutting out ten inches of the sciatic nerve, all tissue around it, making quite a cavity, then covering the whole area with the large muscle taken from the back of Bill's left shoulder—two surgeries. Bill would carry a dead weight, plus, his leg would have no feeling. I thought this would be more difficult than having no leg at all. We were told that sores would develop, plus, live cancer cells would be left in his leg.

A few days later, after letting this sink in, with careful wording, I asked, "Wouldn't this be the time to amputate? I don't think we should mess around anymore; what do you think, Bill?"

That was easy for me to say. It wasn't my leg.

Bill wanted to go slow. "Let's have the surgery first and go from there."

I understood his decision, but back home, after telling our grown children, they all agreed taking the leg off at this time was the better decision. I prayed that my dear husband could make this change in his life by deciding to walk into the hospital and come out in a wheelchair, having one leg. It wasn't long before he agreed losing the leg was better than keeping it. I was thankful but afraid.

How will this affect him? How will this affect me? Our life will be different. "Okay, God, lead and guide us; please help us get through this change and help us grow." This was heavy.

Back down to Houston on June 18, 2019. Surgery was on June 20th. We prayed, we talked, we felt the love of God. From the beginning, we felt carried. We still do. I've had peace in my soul, and that is from the love and prayers of many, for which I am forever thankful. I'm in awe of all the prayers that are sent up on our behalf. It's a lesson in my prayer life—to be more diligent and to spend more time in loving those I love and care about, including humanity across this world, all loved by our Lord. We all need prayer; we all have challenges in life, each and every one.

My Bill was wheeled off to have his right leg cut off. *Is this real? How did we get here?* I had faith and hope and peace in my heart. I was ready; Bill was ready. I thought, *He's losing a leg, but he has the rest of his earthly body; he is alive.*

We are so blessed. There is always someone less fortunate, always.

I was floating. The six hours went by quickly, and the doctor was ready to talk. "I am finished; everything went well!"

"Thank you for caring for my husband." I wondered, "Why am I blessed to hear those words, Lord? Thank you for loving and caring for my Bill."

It's all in His plan. Right then, this was our plan.

I was able to go to recovery then. There he was, awake but groggy. I greeted him with a hug and kisses, tears too. I didn't look past his chest, afraid to look, but after my tentative weirdness, I looked, and I saw only one leg.

Wow, can I do this? Can we do this? Yes, we can do this! It's not more than we can handle; we aren't alone.

Bill spent six days in the hospital, and while there, our three daughters flew down to see their father and just be with their mother for support. It was a great gift! Thank you Erin, Macy, and Molly!

We then spent two weeks at our hotel, close to the hospital, to heal and rest, to learn, and to have physical therapy and acupuncture for phantom pain. It was a long three weeks but a good time to become accustomed to and accept our new way of life. It felt good being the nurse— taking care of meds, figuring out a walker and wheelchair and how to navigate the handicap bathroom, shower, and toilet. We got out of the room as much as we could but spent most of our days in the hotel and hospital combined. Wheeling everywhere, checking out shops, and getting snacks and eating was the best pastime. Then we came back to the room for rest, lots of rest. I slept a lot myself from days prior, healing from anxiety and worry. Rest was the best medicine.

Let's go home—but how do we navigate with one leg into a van, wheelchair into airport, get into the plane seat, bathroom?

Everything had to be thought out—be prepared, be flexible, be kind, be patient. It was our new us. It was better if we worked together; there was less frustration. Slow down; do it with thought the first time.

Erin and Ross picked us up in St. Louis. This gave us only one airport to deal with. It was great to be going home after this adventure. Bill was a fantastic patient. I was very proud of his good attitude and demeanor. They were all sad to see him go home, the hospital and hotel, really! He got the "best patient award" from everyone.

We were home a few days, and Bill finally broke down. "It is all real; it happened." Life was different for him how.

I held him, telling him he had to reach this point in healing. He was saying goodbye to life before, saying goodbye to his leg. It made me cry, too.

When we came home, our house was very busy; family and friends stopped by, our kids and grandkids loving on Grandpa and Grandma. We were home! Bill had ups and downs, but he was strong and determined to make it work.

Bill had a setback a couple of weeks ago. He experienced night sweats and fatigue, not feeling well for about a week. After tests and talking with his doctor, we found he had pneumonia and blood clots in his lungs, veins, and artery. He took an antibiotic and had to take a blood thinner to dissolve the clots, two daily shots administered in his abdomen by himself for three months or longer. I was thankful he didn't mind doing it himself. That is not my thing! We canceled our trip down to Houston to pick up his new leg. Bill was too weak and tired from pneumonia. Our plan was to go back the end of October. We prayed it was a good fit, comfortable and safe, to give him more freedom in getting around without the aid of the walker, wheelchair, or crutches.

These words tell my side of the story—what I felt while he went though the past eight years, having three tumors removed from his right leg, one at a time, to the amputation of that leg. We are making it, with some days of confusion. "What should I do? Where do I go from here?" God is with us each day, leading us forward. All we need do is believe and follow Him.

I love you, Bill Mayo, and pray for many more years with you! God bless you and keep you safe, healthy, and happy!

EPILOGUE

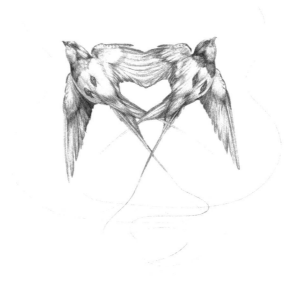

EILEEN

There is one more character to reveal—not in the sense of a cast member but in the sense of an attribute. Yes, it's *Eileen*. Perhaps it's but another shameless attempt at humor, but I think it's more than that. I specifically chose this name for the epilogue because I could not have made it this far through the Stanley saga unless I *leaned*. Throughout this entire trek, I've been leaning. I've leaned on my wife, my family, my friends, my medical team, and most certainly, I've leaned on Howard. Even when I didn't know

He was there, His quiet presence provided stability for my footsteps. Now, with but one limb, I await His timing on when I might be fitted with a prosthetic leg. But even then, I'll be leaning.

Just recently, for example, Howard has redirected me to a new prosthetist - Mr. David Rotter - in Joliet, Illinois. Dave is a mere two hours from home, and is also a renowned hip disarticulation specialist. Dave does his work as a labor of love, and as Howard continues His loving work, I will continue to lean.

People have asked me, "What are your main takeaways from this journey with Stanley?" They are manifold and difficult to distill. Clearly, Howard has been working on me spiritually for years. Long before Stanley and long after, I trust. Through Stanley, He's taught me several notable lessons.

Perhaps number one would be this—as I've said before, I firmly believe Howard did not *allow* Stanley to occur. He directed Stanley to occur. My first cancer—*self*—had to be confronted. What better means than to strip away the façade of my own making, placing me in circumstances of utter vulnerability and dependence upon so many others? Howard was clearly taking this hard-headed pupil to school. He also provided a steady stream of *Howard Moments* along the way—evidence of His working, both prominently and quietly behind the scenes, orchestrating the many outcomes of the Stanley saga. To deny that He directed the entire voyage is incomprehensible to me. There's just no other satisfactory explanation. He was teaching me, teaching me to *lean—on Him and on those I love.*

Takeaway number two would have to be the lessons I've learned about prayer. Of course, (and due to my not-quite-dormant pride), I'd like to think there has been a lot of spiritual growth in me as a result of Stanley. Maybe you'll forgive this as boasting in the Lord and not in myself. Before Stanley, I could not have been called a prayer warrior. Not even close. In fact, I prayed rather inconsistently and selfishly, calling upon Howard only when it suited me or when I wanted something. I've certainly come to rely upon and recognize the power of prayer. Not for my selfish wants and needs but as a means of worship and communion with Him. Prayer permits us to encounter God, to draw near to Him, and enables His grace to transform us. It will strip away our false illusions of significance, power, and arrogant self-reliance.

I've changed my own habits from merely saying, "I'll pray for you," as a casual utterance to immediately acting upon that expression and actually praying, right then and there. I've learned, too, that I need prayer. Prayers sustained both Gail and me during our days of challenge and struggle, and I'm more keenly aware that I am not alone in that need. My children, their spouses, my grandkids, my friends, our government leaders, and our nation— *All* need prayer. It is not something *nice to do*; it is something Christians are called to do.

We all have our baggage, and we do not have to carry our baggage alone. Cancer is just another form of baggage. Jesus says in Matthew 11:29-30, "Take my yoke upon you, and learn of me; for I am meek and lowly in heart: and ye shall find rest unto your souls. For my yoke *is* easy, and my burden is light."

Howard carried us. And Howard will carry you—**If** you allow Him to. In my case, cancer cannot and does not have the last word. Howard does. He eases my worry. He lessens my struggles. He carries my load and will also carry all of your burdens. All you have to do is ask Him.

The third takeaway is the reminder of God's daily presence— those *Howard Moments* that I so often encountered. I've always enjoyed an ironic twist in any story, and Howard was definitely speaking my language—using both irony and subtle humor to relate to me as His unique creation—precisely where I was—as only He could.

God spoke, not in an audible voice, of course, but through the many marvelous revelations of His choreography. His perfect sense of irony and awesome sense of humor were powerful throughout my experience. How ironic that I once believed I was *three people*—who I thought I was, who I wanted others to think I am, and who I really am. *I've learned that no one can pull off the Trinity, except God*. Also, a trinity of hospital stays stripped away my false sense of self-sufficiency, replacing it with a whole person, redeemed and accepted as a son by our Heavenly Father. It also took three surgeries to eradicate Stanley. How ironic that he, too, started out as a *tough guy* but ultimately yielded to Howard and capable medical intervention. Howard's presence is a common thread throughout my trek. And I love that He spoke to me in ways that I could not deny His company!

Perhaps the final takeaway I'll relate is this. No matter how self-reliant we think we are in this life, we are not sufficient apart from God. He made us. He made us for His pleasure and for His glory. He desires communion and fellowship with us. As tough-minded as we might think we are, we cannot muscle through life. We are not in control, and we desperately need Howard. Stanley's residence allowed Howard to show me how temporal life is. And how our concentrated focus needs to shift from the temporal to the eternal. Ecclesiastes 12:13 sums it up nicely: "Let us hear the conclusion of the whole matter: Fear God, and keep his commandments: for this *is* the whole *duty* of man."

Thus far, through the Stanley experience, I have survived. I might go so far as to say I have thrived. I am a far stronger Christian today because of Stanley. It is so true that Howard's strength is perfected in my weakness. I'm thankful to know that He is still very much with me now—bearing me up and loving me as only He can. Reflecting on my life's journey, I'll have to admit that although I was saved at sixteen, I didn't become a committed follower of Christ until my fifties—until *Stanley*. Stiff-necked and proud, I wandered in my own wilderness for over forty years.

I'm not sure what the future holds. Negative margins are a good thing following amputation. But, as the medical team warned, it does not mean that Stanley might not rear his ornery head some-place else. None of us are promised tomorrow, but I like Miles Davis's quote: "My future starts when I wake up every morning." (Davis, Miles, and Quincy Troupe. *Miles.* New York: Simon and Schuster Paperbacks, 2005)

For the time Howard has left for me, I want to proclaim that Stanley was indeed a gift. I won't waste this gift but will use it to glorify God. Yes, of course, I realize that I was in the hands of some very gifted physicians over the course of the past many years. I celebrate their gifts, much as we all admire and celebrate any special talent of individuals who use and display them.

But how many times do we applaud the *Gift-giver*? That's Howard. As thankful as I was for the special skills of my medical team, I celebrate and praise the Gift-giver—the Great Physician, *Howard*, who bestowed those talents upon them.

With a final nod to Gail, I should mention my answer when asked if I have any regrets. The context of that question is always my amputation. Did I have any regrets about pursuing the ampu-tation path? The simple answer to that question is, no. I don't have any regrets about that at all. It's a hill I will climb. I do think some things are regrettable regarding cancer in this country, and I believe Gail is on the right track.

I don't think diet would have prevented Stanley because as I've said, Stanley was Howard's gift to me. But I do have to agree with Gail that in today's world, we eat too much crap. Fast food, soda, and chemically-laced and processed food that in many cases has been stripped of any nutritional value. We hear a lot about health care in the news and in political discourse these days, but the truth is, they're not really talking about health care.

I was sucked into that medical vortex for the past eight years— up close and personal. Not once did we discuss health care. We always discussed disease management. Truth is, we don't have a health care system; we have a disease management system. What we put in our bellies contributes, I'm certain, to the rampant disease so prevalent in our nation. We definitely need to focus more on disease prevention—true health care—and less on disease management. There are signs that medical doctors and the universities that train them are becoming more aware of the connection between lifestyle and cancer. We are accountable for our choices, and we are responsible for our own physical health.

Our body is the temple of God. We need to be mindful of that every day. It is, again, as are all things in this temporal life, a gift from Howard. The strong relationship between what we consume and our physical well-being likewise extends to our spiritual life. What we consume mentally and emotionally is inextricably linked to our spiritual well-being. I know. I came close to derailment many times due to what I was consuming intellectually. There is no shortage of spiritual *junk food*. My urging to all is to feast instead upon God's True Word. From His Word comes the fulness of life that each of us seeks. Psalm 16:11 comes to mind, "Thou wilt shew me the path of life: in my presence is fulness of joy; at thy right hand there are pleasures for evermore."

Finally, if you've read this over-the-shoulder look at my past eight-year journey with Stanley, thank you. Thank you for allowing me to tell my story. It has been therapeutic for me, and I pray that it has been uplifting to you. Remember this excerpt from Romans 5, verses 2 through 5: "...we rejoice in hope of the glory of God. More than that, we rejoice in our sufferings, knowing that suffering produces endurance, and endurance produces character, and character produces hope, and hope does not put us to shame, because God's love has been poured into our hearts through the Holy Spirit who has been given to us."

Howard is available to each one of us. He issues an invitation through His Word. My prayer is for everyone to walk with Howard.

He has a plan, and He has it covered. And no evil that befalls man is greater than He.

In the final book of the Bible, Revelation tells us that we are saved by the grace of God and our Lord Jesus Christ. This is the truth that contains the ultimate solution to any struggle, any problem. We simply must: **A**cknowledge that we are sinners and need a Savior, **B**elieve that Jesus Christ is our Savior and that we need Him, and **C**onfess Him as Lord of our life. As simple as A, B, C. If you look for Howard, you'll find Him. He is never far away. And He desires that you lean on Him.

THE END

APPENDIX

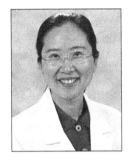

Dr. Jane Liu, Oncology, Illinois Cancer Care

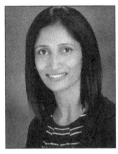

Dr. Neeta Somaiha, Sarcoma Medical Oncology. M.D. Anderson

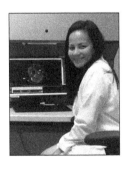

Dr. Keila Torres, Surgical Oncology. M.D. Anderson

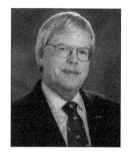

Dr. Stanley Hamilton, Pathology & Laboratory Medicine M.D. Anderson

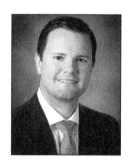

Dr. Alexander Mericli, Reconstruction Surgery M.D. Anderson

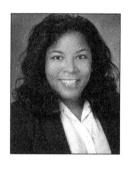

Dr. Valerae Lewis, Chief of Orthopedic Oncology M.D. Anderson

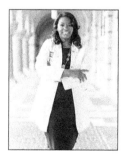

Dr. Alysia Kemp, Orthopedic Oncology Fellow M.D. Anderson

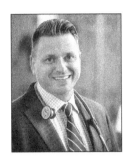

Dr. Trent Proehl, Medical Arts, Tremont, IL

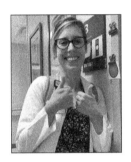

Nadia Leach, Physician's Assistant, Orthopedics, M.D. Anderson

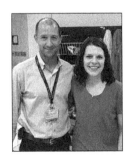

Mr. Alex Penny & Ms. Leslie Ott, Physical & Occupational Therapy, M.D. Anderson

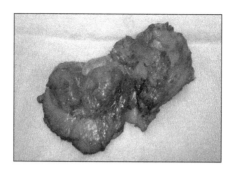

Stanley, after first resection (February 2012)

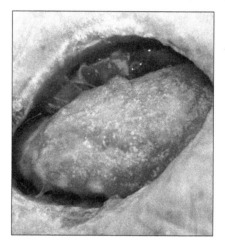

Stanley's initial wound after eight months (June 2012)

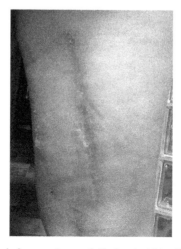

Stanley's former home fully healed (April 2013)

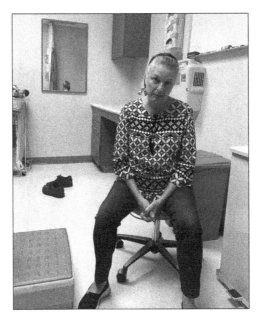

Gail, upon learning of First Cousin Stanley's Return (August 2017)

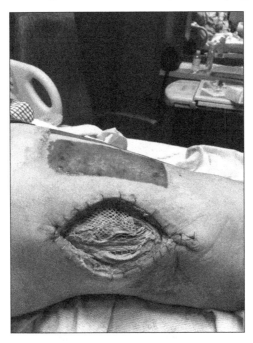

Second surgery, First Cousin Stanley's Removal (October 2017)

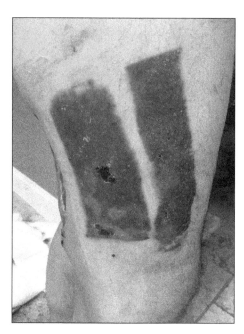

Skin graft for First Cousin Stanley (October 2017)

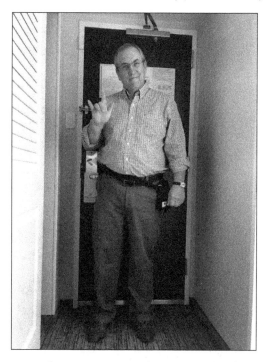

Leaving for amputation surgery, Second Cousin Stanley (June 20th, 2019)

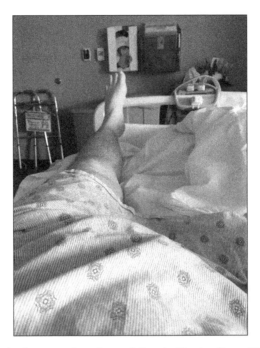

My first look – me minus Second Cousin Stanley (June 20, 2019)

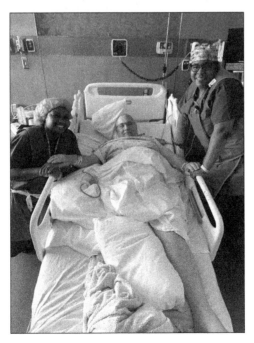

Dr. Kemp (l) and Dr. Lewis – day one minus Stanley (June 21st, 2019)

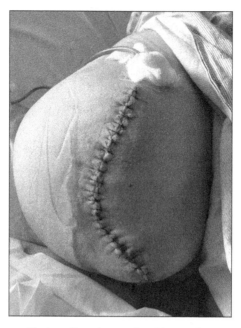

Some nifty handiwork – or should I say "legwork"?

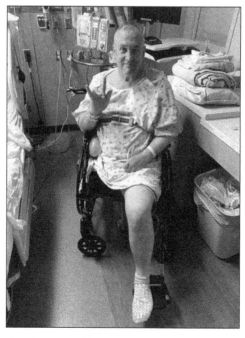

First time out of bed post-surgery (June 2019)

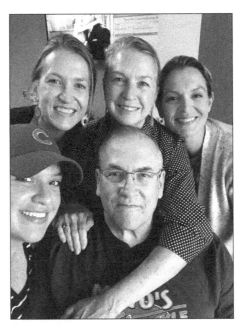

My post-surgical support team (l-r): Molly, Erin, Gail, Macy (June 2019)

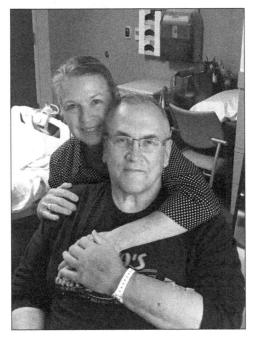

Gail and me on Discharge Day (June 27th, 2019)

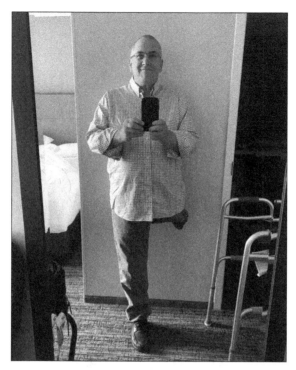

Out on the town post-surgery (June 30th, 2019)

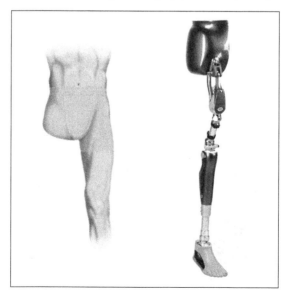

What comes next? My new "Joint Venture!"

My new Best Friends

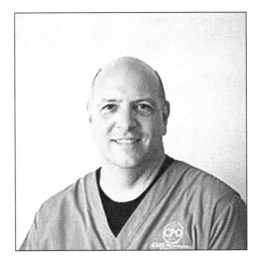

Mr. Dave Baty, Care Prosthetics & Orthotics, Houston, TX

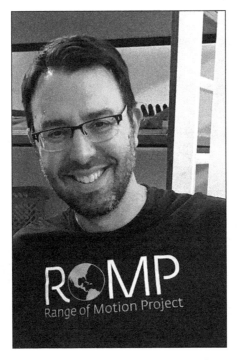

Mr. David Rotter, Rotter Prosthetics, Joliet, IL

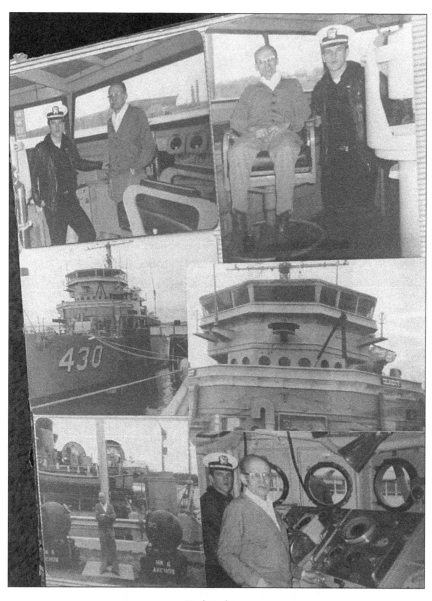

Dad and me

CPSIA information can be obtained
at www.ICGtesting.com
Printed in the USA
BVHW022014030220
571297BV00001B/1